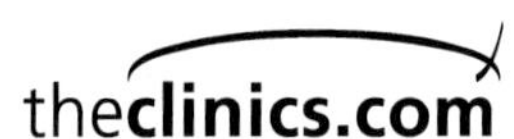
theclinics.com

ORTHOPEDIC CLINICS
OF NORTH AMERICA

Elbow Trauma

GUEST EDITOR
Scott P. Steinmann, MD

April 2008 • Volume 39 • Number 2

SAUNDERS

An Imprint of Elsevier, Inc.
PHILADELPHIA   LONDON   TORONTO   MONTREAL   SYDNEY   TOKYO

W.B. SAUNDERS COMPANY

A Division of Elsevier Inc.

Elsevier Inc., 1600 John F. Kennedy Blvd., Suite 1800, Philadelphia, PA 19103-2899.

http://www.orthopedic.theclinics.com

ORTHOPEDIC CLINICS OF NORTH AMERICA
April 2008
Editor: Debora Dellapena

Volume 39, Number 2
ISSN 0030-5898
ISBN-10: 1-4160-5817-6
ISBN-13: 978-1-4160-5817-5

Orthopedic Clinics of North America (ISSN 0030-5898) is published quarterly (For Post Office use only: Volume 39 issue 1 of 4) by Elsevier Inc., 360 Park Avenue South, New York, NY 10010-1710. Months of publication are January, April, July, and October. Business and Editorial Offices: 1600 John F. Kennedy Blvd., Suite 1800, Philadelphia, PA 19103-2899. Customer Service Office: 6277 Sea Harbor Drive, Orlando, FL 33887-4800. Periodicals postage paid at New York, NY and additional mailing offices. Subscription prices are $226.00 per year for (US individuals), $389.00 per year for (US institutions), $267.00 per year (Canadian individuals), $456.00 per year (Canadian institutions), $309.00 per year (international individuals), $456.00 per year (international institutions), $113.00 per year (US students), $154.00 per year (Canadian and international students). Foreign air speed delivery is included in all *Clinics* subscription prices. All prices are subject to change without notice. **POSTMASTER:** Send address changes to *Orthopedic Clinics of North America*, Elsevier Periodicals Customer Service, 6277 Sea Harbor Drive, Orlando, FL 32887-4800. **Customer Service: 1-800-654-2452 (US). From outside the United States, call 1-407-563-6020. Fax: 1-407-363-9661. E-mail: JournalsCustomerService-usa@elsevier.com.**

Reprints. For copies of 100 or more, of articles in this publication, please contact the Commercial Reprints Department, Elsevier Inc., 360 Park Avenue South, New York, New York 10010-1710. Tel. (212) 633-3813, Fax: (212) 462-1935, E-mail: reprints@elsevier.com.

Orthopedic Clinics of North America is covered in *Index Medicus, Cinahl, Excerpta Medica, and Cumulative Index to Nursing and Allied Health Literature.*

Printed in the United States of America.

GUEST EDITOR

SCOTT P. STEINMANN, MD, Associate Professor of Orthopedic Surgery, Department of Orthopedic Surgery, Mayo Clinic, Rochester, Minnesota

CONTRIBUTORS

ROBERT A. ARCIERO, MD, Professor, Department of Orthopaedic Surgery, University of Connecticut, John Dempsey Hospital, Farmington, Connecticut

APRIL D. ARMSTRONG, BSc(PT), MD, MSc, FRCSC, Associate Professor, Department of Orthopaedics and Rehabilitation, Penn State College of Medicine, Penn State Milton S. Hershey Medical Center, Hershey, Pennsylvania

GEORGE S. ATHWAL, MD, FRCSC, Assistant Professor of Surgery; Consultant, Hand and Upper Limb Centre, St. Joseph's Health Care, University of Western Ontario, London, Ontario, Canada

CHRIS D. BRYCE, MD, Resident in Orthopaedic Surgery, Department of Orthopaedics and Rehabilitation, Penn State College of Medicine, Penn State Milton S. Hershey Medical Center, Hershey, Pennsylvania

EMILIE V. CHEUNG, MD, Assistant Professor, Orthopaedic Surgery, Stanford University Hospital and Clinics, Stanford, California

KENNETH J. FABER, MD, MHPE, FRCSC, Associate Professor of Surgery; Consultant, Hand and Upper Limb Centre, St. Joseph's Health Care, University of Western Ontario, London, Ontario, Canada

LARRY D. FIELD, MD, Fellow, Upper Extremity Service, Mississippi Sports Medicine and Orthopaedic Center; Clinical Instructor, Department of Orthopaedic Surgery, University of Mississippi School of Medicine, Jackson, Mississippi

THOMAS J. GOETZ, MD, FRCSC, Assistant Professor of Orthopedics, Department of Orthopedics, St. Paul's Hospital, University of British Columbia, Vancouver, British Columbia, Canada

SEAN P. GRACE, MD, Fellow, Mississippi Sports Medicine and Orthopaedic Center, Jackson, Mississippi

MARK JENSEN, MD, Resident in General Surgery, Department of General Surgery, Mayo Clinic, Rochester, Minnesota

MICHAEL A. KUHN, MD, Naval Hospital Camp Lejeune, Department of Orthopaedics, Camp Lejeune, North Carolina

AUGUSTUS D. MAZZOCCA, MD, Assistant Professor, Department of Orthopaedic Surgery, University of Connecticut, John Dempsey Hospital, Farmington, Connecticut

STEVEN L. MORAN, MD, Associate Professor, Division of Plastic Surgery; Department of Orthopedic Surgery, Mayo Clinic, Rochester, Minnesota

J. WHITCOMB POLLOCK, MD, FRCSC, Clinical Fellow, Hand and Upper Limb Centre, St. Joseph's Health Care, University of Western Ontario, London, Ontario, Canada

YISHAI ROSENBLATT, MD, Clinical Fellow, Hand and Upper Limb Centre, St. Joseph's Health Care, University of Western Ontario, London, Ontario, Canada

GLEN ROSS, MD, Department of Orthopaedics and Sports Medicine, Orthopaedic Sports Medicine, New England Baptist Hospital, Boston, Massachusetts

M. WADE SHRADER, MD, The CORE Institute, Phoenix, Arizona

JEFFREY T. SPANG, MD, Sports Medicine Fellow, Department of Orthopaedic Surgery, University of Connecticut, John Dempsey Hospital, Farmington, Connecticut

SCOTT P. STEINMANN, MD, Department of Orthopedic Surgery, Mayo Clinic, Rochester, Minnesota

CHRISTIAN J.H. VEILLETTE, MD, MSc, FRCSC, Department of Orthopedic Surgery, Mayo Clinic, Rochester, Minnesota

CONTRIBUTORS

CONTENTS

Preface   ix
Scott P. Steinmann

Anatomy and Biomechanics of the Elbow   141
Chris D. Bryce and April D. Armstrong

> The elbow is a complex, highly constrained joint that provides critical range of motion to the upper extremity needed for performing the normal activities of daily living. The elbow is protected by a fortress of individual static and dynamic constraints that function together to provide stability. Knowing the identity and specific functions of each stabilizing structure facilitates appropriate diagnosis and treatment of the acutely injured elbow.

Acute Elbow Dislocations   155
Michael A. Kuhn and Glen Ross

> The elbow is the second most commonly dislocated major joint in the adult age group and the most commonly dislocated major joint in the pediatric population. The mechanism of injury and resultant ligamentous disruption pattern have been investigated and noted. Classification of elbow dislocation is well described, and allows for appropriate treatment and rehabilitation. For stable reductions, an aggressive early ROM protocol emphasizing active motion has been helpful for maximizing final range of motion and minimizing extension loss. Associated injuries with elbow dislocation are common and can result in significant morbidity if not diagnosed and treated.

Pediatric Supracondylar Fractures and Pediatric Physeal Elbow Fractures   163
M. Wade Shrader

> Elbow fractures in children are extremely common, making up approximately 15% of all fractures in pediatric patients. The unique radiographic anatomy of the pediatric elbow, along with the potential for neurovascular compromise, often provokes anxiety in orthopedic surgeons. A thorough understanding of the anatomy and treatment principles makes the care for these children more straightforward, however. The distal humerus makes up approximately 85% of all elbow fractures in children. The most common fractures of the distal humerus in children are supracondylar humerus fractures, lateral condyle fractures, medial epicondyle fractures, and transphyseal humerus fractures. Each of these fractures is discussed in detail, outlining their radiographic features, principles of treatment, and potential complications.

Current Recommendations for the Treatment of Radial Head Fractures   **173**
Yishai Rosenblatt, George S. Athwal, and Kenneth J. Faber

> Radial head fractures are the most common type of elbow fractures. Although a consensus has emerged that favors the nonsurgical treatment of undisplaced fractures, controversy surrounds the treatment of displaced radial head fractures. Further research is necessary to provide a better scientific rationale for making treatment recommendations. Options for the treatment of displaced fractures include nonoperative management, fragment excision, whole head excision, open reduction and internal fixation, and radial head arthroplasty. The purpose of this article is to review the mechanisms that result in radial head fracture, to describe important physical findings that assist in identifying injuries associated with radial head fractures, and to define the role of the various interventions described for the treatment of radial head fractures.

Distal Humerus Fractures   **187**
J. Whitcomb Pollock, Kenneth J. Faber, and George S. Athwal

> Intra-articular fractures of the distal humerus are among the most challenging fractures to manage. Nonoperative treatment, although appropriate for some patients, often leads to loss of motion and unsatisfactory functional outcomes. Over the last 2 decades, enhanced operative techniques and implant designs have improved the reduction and stability of distal humerus fractures leading to better outcomes. Careful preoperative planning, adequate exposure, and stable fixation facilitating early mobilization are essential to achieve successful outcomes with internal fixation.

Prosthetic Replacement for Distal Humerus Fractures   **201**
George S. Athwal, Thomas J. Goetz, J. Whitcomb Pollock, and Kenneth J. Faber

> Primary total elbow arthroplasty is a treatment option for elderly patients with osteopenic bone, increased comminution, and articular fragmentation. Recently, there has been a renewed interest in distal humerus hemiarthroplasty for the treatment of distal humerus fractures, including coronal shear fractures of the capitellum and trochlea. This article focuses on the evaluation and management of distal humerus fractures with prosthetic replacement.

Chronic Medial Elbow Instability   **213**
Sean P. Grace and Larry D. Field

> Chronic medial elbow instability can be a debilitating problem for the throwing athlete. It affects non-throwers much less commonly regarding activities of daily living. Instability can occur as a result of repetitive microtrauma over a long period of time or as a result of a single traumatic event. If left untreated, the resulting sequelae can lead to chronic pain, ulnar neuritis, and inability to compete/work.

Chronic Lateral Elbow Instability   **221**
Emilie V. Cheung

> Posterolateral rotatory instability of the elbow is the most common pattern of chronic lateral elbow instability. The primary lesion in posterolateral rotatory instability is injury

CONTENTS

or attenuation of the lateral ulnar collateral ligament. Posterolateral rotatory instability is diagnosed on the basis of careful history taking and specific physical examination techniques. Reconstruction of the lateral ulnar collateral ligament with repair of the surrounding soft tissue structures is recommended in patients who have symptoms of recurrent lateral instability. Open and arthroscopic reconstruction techniques have resulted in improvement of elbow function and satisfactory results in most patients, although mild limitation in terminal extension of the elbow is a common finding.

Olecranon Fractures   229
Christian J.H. Veillette and Scott P. Steinmann

Approximately 10% of fractures about the adult elbow consist of fractures of the olecranon process of the ulna and range from simple nondisplaced fractures to complex fracture–dislocations of the elbow. Several treatment options for internal fixation have been described, including tension-band wiring, plate fixation, intramedullary screw fixation, and triceps advancement after fragment excision. The method of internal fixation is chosen based primarily on fracture type. Because olecranon fractures are all intra-articular injuries, they require anatomic or essentially normal surface reduction and trochlear notch contour for predictable outcomes. In addition, fixation must be stable enough to permit early mobilization to avoid significant elbow stiffness. Given the variability in fracture patterns, the complex anatomy, and associated injuries, treating surgeons must be familiar with multiple treatment methods and follow a systematic surgical strategy to avoid complications and achieve reliable outcomes.

Distal Biceps Rupture   237
Augustus D. Mazzocca, Jeffrey T. Spang, and Robert A. Arciero

Recognition and treatment of distal biceps tendon ruptures is increasing, likely because of greater clinical awareness and the greater activity and demands of the middle-aged population. This article focuses on the proper evaluation and treatment of distal biceps tendon ruptures with special attention focused on recently developed techniques. A review of the recent clinical literature will accompany an overview of pertinent biomechanical studies and an explanation of the risks and benefits of the most popular surgical techniques for distal biceps repair.

Soft Tissue Coverage of the Elbow: A Reconstructive Algorithm   251
Mark Jensen and Steven L. Moran

Soft tissue defects can occur for various reasons, but they are primarily due to trauma, tumor, and infection. Coverage choices may include primary closure, skin grafting, local cutaneous flaps, fasciocutaneous transposition flaps, island fascial or fasciocutaneous flaps, muscle or myocutaneous pedicled flaps, and microvascular free-tissue transfer. Despite the multitude of options for coverage, the authors have found four flaps to provide reliable coverage for most elbow deficits within their practice; these flaps are the latissimus dorsi flap, the radial forearm flap, the anconeus flap, and the free anterior lateral thigh flap. This article provides an overview of treatment options for elbow coverage, with specific emphasis on the use of these four specific flaps.

Index   265

FORTHCOMING ISSUES

July 2008

Patellofemoral Arthritis
Wayne B. Leadbetter, MD,
Guest Editor

October 2008

Shoulder Trauma
George S. Athwal, MD, FRCSC,
Guest Editor

January 2009

Spine Oncology
Rakesh R. Donthineni, MD,
Guest Editor

RECENT ISSUES

January 2008

**Orthopedic Ancillary Services:
A Guide to Practice Management**
Jack M. Bert, MD,
Guest Editor

October 2007

Scoliosis
Anthony A. Stans, MD,
Guest Editor

July 2007

Minimally Invasive Spine Surgery
Dino Samartzis, DSc, MSc, Dip EBHC,
Francis H. Shen, MD,
D. Greg Anderson, MD,
Guest Editors

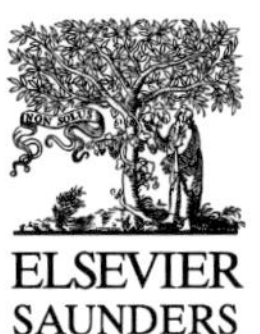

ELSEVIER
SAUNDERS

Orthop Clin N Am 39 (2008) ix

ORTHOPEDIC
CLINICS
OF NORTH AMERICA

Preface

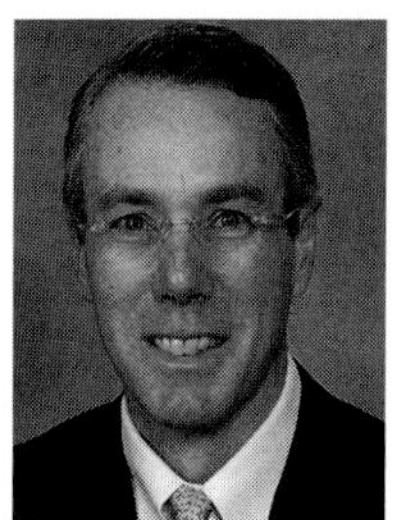

Scott P. Steinmann, MD
Guest Editor

This issue of *Orthopedic Clinics of North America* is devoted to the treatment of elbow trauma. Treating elbow trauma has been of significant interest over the past few years. Much has changed in the operative and non-operative approach to the traumatized elbow. The use of improved imaging techniques, such as 3-D computerized tomography, has also allowed us to better understand the basic fracture patterns of the humerus, ulna, and radius.

This greater ability to visualize the fracture has changed our approach to treatment algorithms. Surgical management has become more commonplace; the "bag-of-bones" approach has all but disappeared. Investigators have begun to seriously study the effects of surgical treatment of elbow trauma. Presumed gold standards of treatment are now being subjected to scientific standards of review.

There have been several biomechanical studies over the past few years, which have helped guide us in the choice of treatment options. New reports on fixation techniques of several of the common types of elbow injuries have appeared recently in the literature.

The advances in technology that have occurred in orthopedic trauma care have benefited the treatment of patients with elbow injuries. It was not that long ago when the hardware available to internally fix elbow fractures was the same as that used for forearm or ankle fractures.

Fracture-specific products now exist for treatment of all aspects of elbow trauma—from biceps ruptures to radial head fractures. It is our responsibility to study the outcomes of treatment to understand if the greater cost of this new innovation truly benefits our patients.

I would like to thank all the authors of this issue who were asked to contribute because of their known expertise on elbow trauma. Also, this edition could not have been completed without the excellent guidance of Debora Dellapena.

Scott P. Steinmann, MD
Department of Orthopedic Surgery
Mayo Clinic
200 First Street, SW
Rochester, MN 55905, USA

E-mail address: Steinmann.Scott@mayo.edu

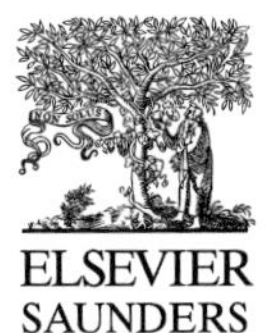

ORTHOPEDIC
CLINICS
OF NORTH AMERICA

Orthop Clin N Am 39 (2008) 141–154

Anatomy and Biomechanics of the Elbow

Chris D. Bryce, MD, April D. Armstrong, BSc(PT), MD, MSc, FRCSC*

*Department of Orthopaedics and Rehabilitation, Penn State College of Medicine,
Penn State Milton S. Hershey Medical Center, H089, 500 University Drive,
P.O. Box 850, Hershey, PA 17033-0850, USA*

A sound understanding of elbow anatomy and biomechanics is necessary to treat common traumatic conditions of the elbow. Combined or isolated injury to vital osseous and soft tissue structures of the elbow joint affects stability. Much work has been accomplished to identify and define the function of the key primary and secondary constraints of the elbow. Biomechanical studies investigating the effect of injury to these structures guide diagnosis and treatment of elbow trauma.

Stability of the elbow is provided by a "fortress" of static and dynamic constraints [1]. The three primary static constraints include the ulnohumeral articulation, the anterior bundle of the medial collateral ligament (MCL), and the lateral collateral ligament (LCL) complex (Fig. 1). If these three structures are intact, the elbow is stable. Secondary constraints include the radiocapitellar articulation, the common flexor tendon, the common extensor tendon, and the capsule. Muscles that cross the elbow joint are the dynamic stabilizers [1]. This article provides a summary of key concepts that are relevant for understanding common elbow injuries. Basic elbow anatomy is presented first, followed by a review of important biomechanical principles.

Elbow anatomy

Osteoarticular anatomy

The articular surfaces of the elbow joint provided by the distal humerus, the proximal

ulna, and the proximal radius are highly irregular and congruent providing inherent osseous stability. The elbow has been called the trochleogingylomoid joint for the hinged (ginglymoid) motion in flexion and extension at the ulnohumeral and radiocapitellar articulations and radial (trochoid) motion in pronation and supination at the proximal radioulnar joint [2].

The distal humerus provides the proximal articular surface of the elbow comprising the trochlea and capitellum (Fig. 2A). The spool-shaped trochlea is centered over the distal humerus in line with the long axis of the humeral shaft. The medial ridge of the trochlea is more prominent than the lateral ridge, which causes 6° to 8° of valgus tilt at its articulation with the greater sigmoid notch of the proximal ulna [3]. The hemispheric-shaped capitellum is lateral to the trochlea and articulates with the concave articular surface of the radial head.

The radial head is important as a secondary stabilizer of the elbow (Fig. 2B). The concave surface of the radial head articulates with the capitellum, whereas the rim of the radial head articulates with the lesser sigmoid notch. Articular cartilage covers the concave surface and an arc of approximately 280° of the rim. Displaced fractures of the radial head can be repaired by screw fixation at the remaining 80° of rim not covered by cartilage [3]. The radial head is not perfectly circular and is variably offset from the axis of the neck, which has important implications in reconstruction of the radial head [4,5].

The highly congruent surfaces of the proximal ulna and trochlea form one of the primary constraints of the elbow joint (Fig. 2C). The sagittal ridge of the greater sigmoid notch runs longitudinally and articulates with the apex of the trochlea.

---

* Corresponding author.

E-mail address: aarmstrong@psu.edu
(A.D. Armstrong).

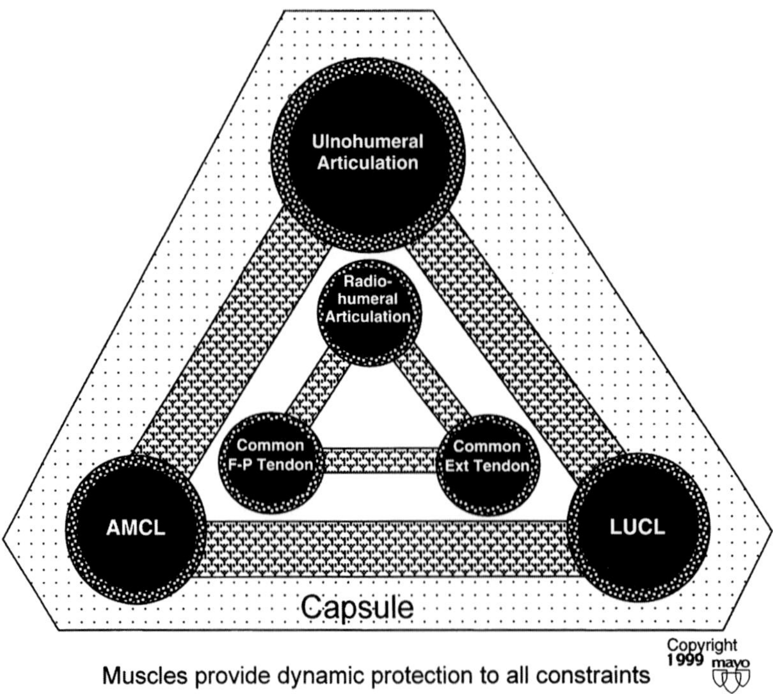

Fig. 1. The "fortress" of static and dynamic constraints to elbow instability. The three primary constraints are the ulnohumeral articulation, the anterior bundle of the medial collateral ligament (AMCL), and the lateral collateral ligament, especially the ulnar part known as the lateral ulnar collateral ligament (LUCL). The secondary constraints are the radiohumeral articulation, the common flexor-pronator (F-P) tendon, the common extensor tendon, and the capsule. The muscles that cross the elbow are the dynamic constraints. (*From* O'Driscoll SW, Jupiter JB, King GJ, et al. The unstable elbow. Instr Course Lect 2001;50:91; with permission.)

The concavities that are medial and lateral to the sagittal ridge complement the convex medial and lateral faces of the trochlea. The lesser sigmoid notch articulates with the rim of the radial head. Osseous stability is enhanced in flexion when the coronoid process locks into the coronoid fossa of the distal humerus, and the radial head is contained in the radial fossa of the distal humerus (see Fig 2A). Osseous stability is enhanced in extension when the tip of the olecranon rotates into the olecranon fossa [6]. The sublime tubercle is the attachment site for the anterior bundle of the MCL.

Capsuloligamentous anatomy

The inherent bony stability together with the capsuloligamentous stabilizers provides the static constraints of the elbow. The static soft tissue stabilizers include the anterior and posterior joint capsule and the medial and LCL complexes. The collateral ligament complexes are medial and lateral capsular thickenings [6].

The capsule attaches along the articular margin of the elbow. The anterior capsule extends proximally above the coronoid and radial fossae, distally to the edge of the coronoid process, and laterally to the annular ligament. The posterior capsule attaches proximally above the olecranon fossa, distally along the medial and lateral articular margins of the greater sigmoid notch, and laterally becomes continuous with the annular ligament. The capsule becomes taut anteriorly when the elbow is extended and posteriorly when the elbow is flexed. Intra-articular pressure is lowest at 70° to 80° of flexion. When fully distended at 80° of flexion, the capacity of the elbow is 25 to 30 mL [7,8]. The capsule provides most of its stabilizing effects with the elbow extended [9].

The MCL complex consists of three components: the anterior bundle or anterior MCL (AMCL), the posterior bundle, and the transverse ligament (Fig. 3). The origin of the MCL is at the anteroinferior surface of the medial epicondyle. The anterior bundle is the most discrete structure

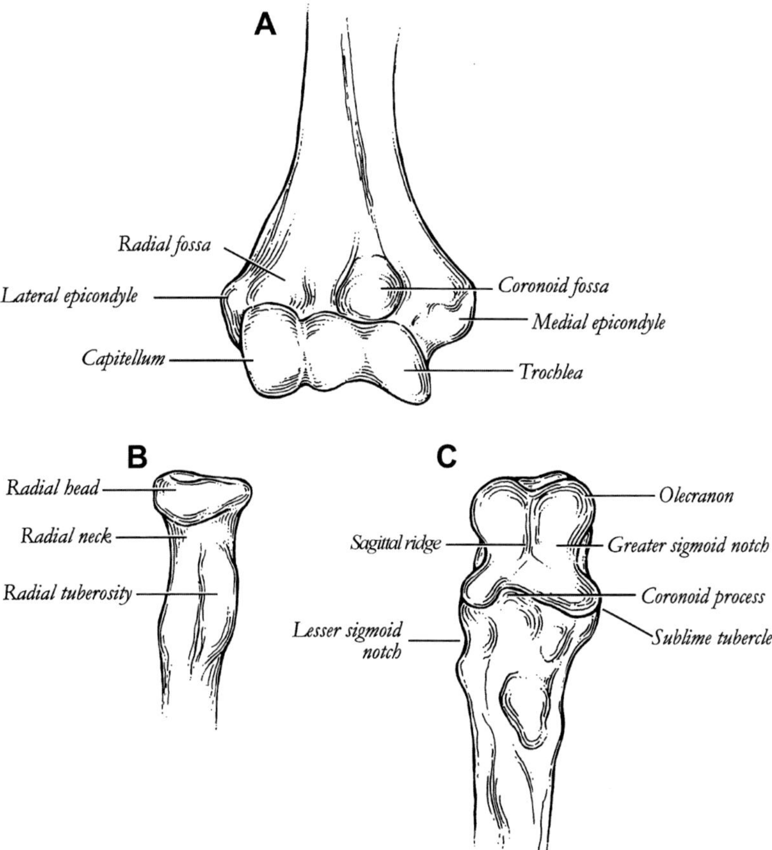

Fig. 2. Osseous elbow anatomy. (*A*) Distal humerus. (*B*) Proximal radius. (*C*) Proximal ulna. (*Adapted from* Armstrong AD, King GJ, Yamaguchi K. Total elbow arthroplasty design. In: Williams GR, Yamaguchi K, Ramsey ML, et al, editors. Shoulder and elbow arthroplasty. Philadelphia: Lippincott Williams & Wilkins; 2005. p. 301; with permission.)

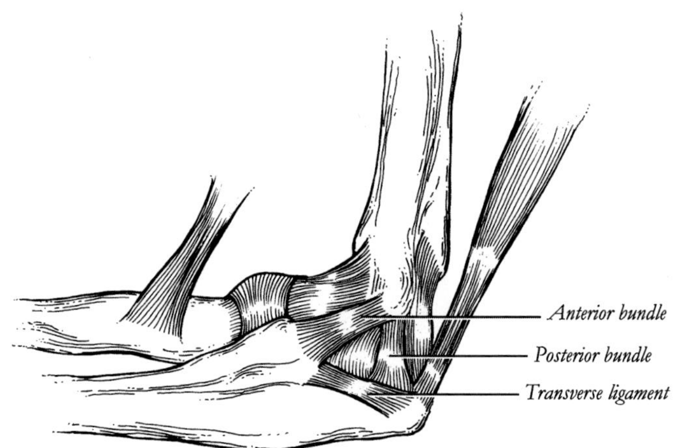

Fig. 3. The medial collateral ligament complex. (*From* Armstrong AD, King GJ, Yamaguchi K. Total elbow arthroplasty design. In: Williams GR, Yamaguchi K, Ramsey ML, et al, editors. Shoulder and elbow arthroplasty. Philadelphia: Lippincott Williams & Wilkins; 2005. p. 303; with permission.)

of the complex and inserts on the anteromedial aspect of the coronoid process, the sublime tubercle. In this position the AMCL is able to provide significant stability against valgus force, making it one of the primary static constraints of the elbow [6]. The anterior bundle is further divided into anterior and posterior bands [10–12]. Some authors include a third central band [13,14]. The posterior bundle is more of a thickening of the capsule rather than a distinct ligament and inserts on the medial olecranon [11]. The transverse ligament runs between the coronoid and the tip of the olecranon and consists of horizontally oriented fibers that often cannot be separated from the capsule. It is believed that the transverse ligament does not contribute significantly to joint stability [12].

The LCL complex consists of four components, including the radial collateral ligament, the lateral ulnar collateral ligament, the annular ligament, and the accessory collateral ligament (Fig. 4). The LCL complex originates along the inferior surface of the lateral epicondyle. The annular ligament attaches to the anterior and posterior margins of the lesser sigmoid notch. The lateral ulnar collateral ligament is one of the primary elbow constraints because it provides varus and posterolateral stability by its insertion distal to the posterior attachment of the annular ligament on the crista supinatoris [15]. The radial collateral ligament inserts into the annular ligament and stabilizes the radial head [6]. The accessory collateral ligament has attachments at the annular ligament and the crista supinatoris.

Muscles

Muscles that cross the elbow joint provide dynamic stabilization to the elbow joint and protect the static constraints. Four groups of muscles cross the elbow: elbow flexors, elbow extensors, forearm flexor-pronators, and forearm extensors. Each muscle that crosses the elbow applies a compressive load to the joint when contracted. Only a few of the muscles that cross the joint act primarily to move the joint, however. The biceps, brachialis, and brachioradialis flex the elbow. The biceps is also the principal supinator of the forearm. The triceps is the main elbow extensor. Although anconeus likely plays a minor role in elbow extension, it is thought to act as a dynamic constraint to varus and posterolateral rotatory instability [6].

Elbow biomechanics

Kinematics

Together with the shoulder, the elbow acts to position the hand in space. Compared to the shoulder, which has a large range of motion in all three axes of rotation, elbow range of motion is relatively constrained.

Flexion-extension

The normal range of elbow motion in flexion and extension is approximately 0° to 140°, with a range of 30° to 130° required for most activities of daily living [16–18]. The flexion-extension axis of the elbow has been described as a loose hinge. Understanding this concept is important in the design and application of endoprostheses, dynamic external fixators, and ligament reconstruction [19–23]. Variation of the flexion axis throughout range of motion is often described in terms of the screw displacement axis (SDA), which shows the

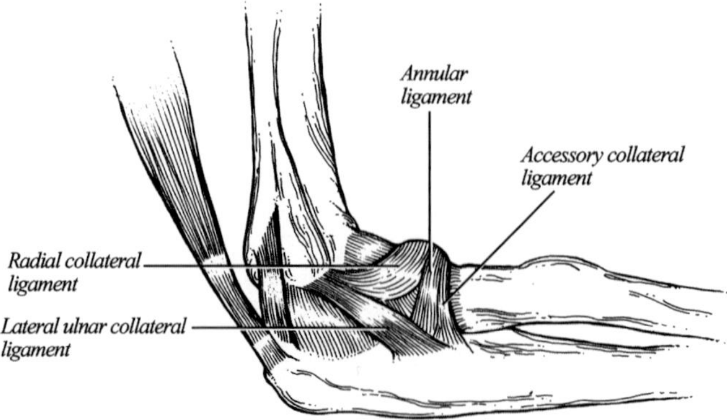

Fig. 4. The lateral collateral ligament complex. (*Adapted from* Armstrong AD, King GJ, Yamaguchi K. Total elbow arthroplasty design. In: Williams GR, Yamaguchi K, Ramsey ML, et al, editors. Shoulder and elbow arthroplasty. Philadelphia: Lippincott Williams & Wilkins; 2005. p. 303; with permission.)

instantaneous rotation and position of the axis throughout flexion. The average SDA has been shown to be in line with the anteroinferior aspect of the medial epicondyle, the center of the trochlea, and the center projection of the capitellum onto a parasagittal plane. One study demonstrated that throughout normal elbow range of motion the instantaneous SDA varies by approximately 3° to 6° in orientation and 1.4 to 2.0 mm in translation [19]. The flexion axis also has been shown to vary with forearm pronation and supination and passive and active movement (Fig. 5) [20]. The average flexion axis of the elbow is oriented at approximately 3° to 5° of internal rotation in relation to the plane of the medial and lateral epicondyles and in 4° to 8° of valgus relative to the long axis of the humerus [6].

Pronation-supination

The radiocapitellar and proximal radioulnar joints of the elbow allow for pronation and supination of the forearm. The normal range of forearm rotation is 180° with pronation of 80° to 90° and supination of approximately 90° [16,24]. Most activities of daily living can be accomplished with 100° of forearm rotation (50° of pronation and 50° of supination) [17]. Although loss of forearm pronation can be compensated to a certain extent by shoulder abduction, there are no effective mechanisms to replace supination [24].

The normal axis of forearm rotation runs from the center of the radial head to the center of the distal ulna [25,26]. It has been stated that axis of rotation is constant and independent of elbow flexion or extension [25]. More recently, however, it

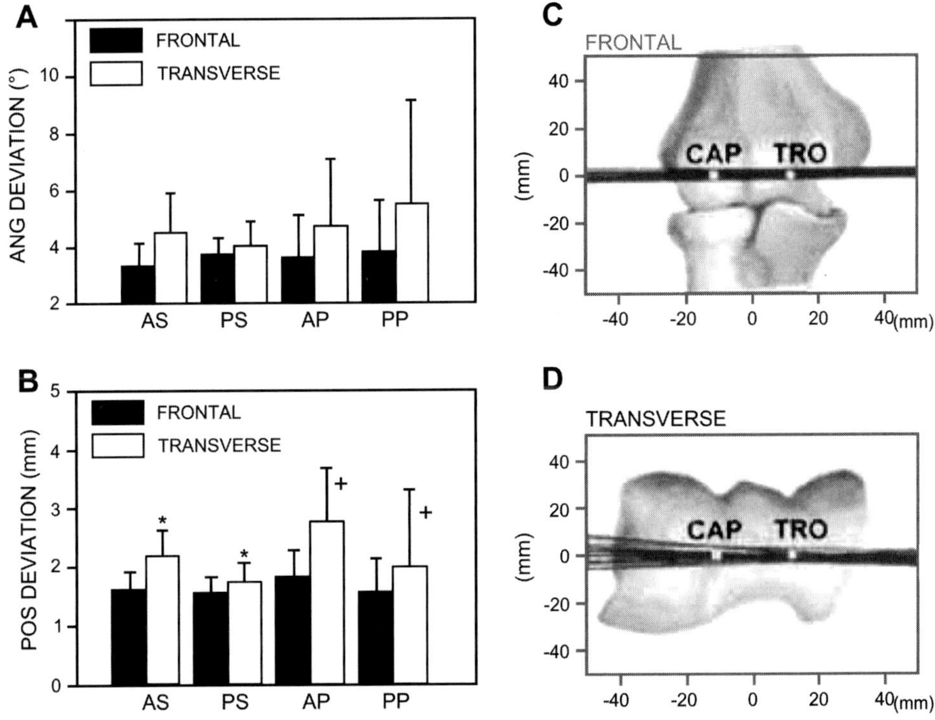

Fig. 5. The flexion axis of the elbow is a loose hinge. The angular (ANG) deviation (*A*) and positional deviation (*B*) for elbow SDAs in the frontal and transverse planes are plotted for the actively and passively flexed elbow with forearm pronation and supination. AS, active supinated; PS, passive supinated; AP, active pronated; PP, passive pronated. Angular deviation is defined as the standard deviation in orientation of all SDAs measured throughout flexion. Positional deviation is defined as the standard deviation in position of all SDAs measured throughout flexion with respect to the humeral origin (the spherical and circular centers of the capitellum and trochlea, respectively). Paired symbols (* and +) represent significant differences. *C* and *D* show the SDAs for a single specimen. CAP, capitellum; TRO, trochlea. (*From* Duck TR, Dunning CE, King GJ, et al. Variability and repeatability of the flexion axis at the ulnohumeral joint. J Orthop Res 2003;21(3):401; with permission.)

was shown that the axis of rotation shifts slightly ulnar and volar during supination and shifts radial and dorsal during pronation [26]. The radius also moves proximally with pronation of the forearm and distally with supination [27].

Forearm rotation plays an important role in stabilizing the elbow, especially when the elbow is moved passively. With passive flexion, the MCL-deficient elbow is more stable in supination, whereas the LCL-deficient elbow is more stable in pronation (Figs. 6 and 7) [28–30]. Research also has shown that the elbow is more stable in supination than in pronation in the setting of coronoid

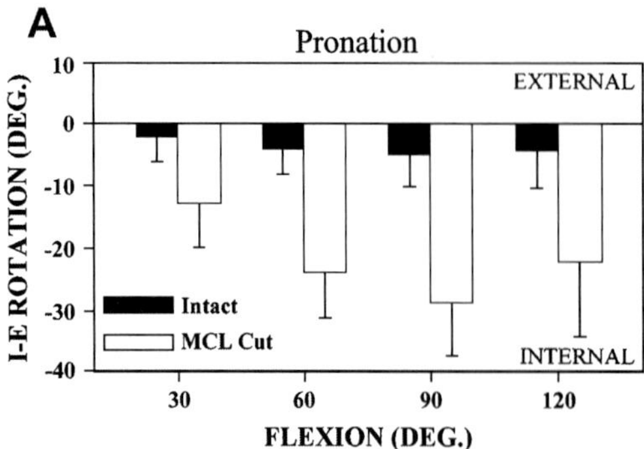

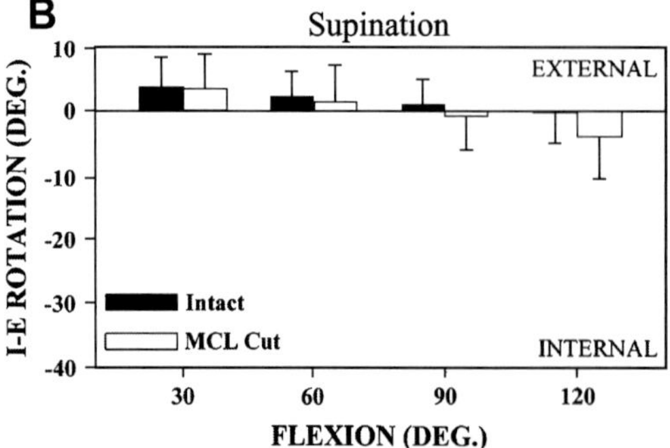

Fig. 6. Passive elbow flexion with the forearm in pronation (*A*) and supination (*B*) for the intact and MCL-deficient elbows. The mean internal-external (I-E) rotation of the ulna with respect to the humerus is plotted for elbow flexion in 30° increments. With the forearm in supination there were no significant differences in I-E rotation between the intact and MCL deficient elbows at 30° and 60° of flexion. There were small but significant differences at 90° and 120°. Overall, for passive flexion of the MCL-deficient elbow there is greater stability with the forearm in supination than in pronation. (*From* Armstrong AD, Dunning CE, Faber KJ, et al. Rehabilitation of the medial collateral ligament-deficient elbow: an in vitro biomechanical study. J Hand Surg [Am] 2000;25(6):1054–5; with permission.)

fractures that involve more than 50% of the coronoid with or without an intact MCL [31]. Another study tested valgus laxity with pronated, supinated, and neutral forearm rotation when the AMCL was intact and severed. It was shown that forearm pronation and supination decreased valgus laxity compared with the neutral forearm position. It was postulated that proximal radial head migration with forearm pronation may increase the joint reaction force at the radiocapitellar articulation, thus increasing valgus elbow stability. It was also hypothesized that increased valgus stability with forearm supination may be the result of increased passive tension in the flexor pronator muscles [32].

Osseous stabilization

The importance of osseous stabilization of the elbow joint is illustrated by the simple (no fractures) elbow dislocation. Most simple elbow dislocations are relatively stable once reduced, although the MCL has been reported to be completely ruptured in nearly all cases and the LCL is disrupted in most cases [33–35]. It has been shown that the congruent articulation of the ulnohumeral joint is responsible for as much as 50% of the stability of the elbow [36].

Coronoid

The coronoid process plays a key role in stabilization of the elbow. Coronoid fractures rarely occur in isolation [37–39]. Some authors have said that a coronoid fracture is pathognomonic for an episode of elbow instability [40]. Fractures of the coronoid are commonly associated with injuries to the collateral ligaments and form part of the definition of the "terrible triad," which is classically defined as an elbow dislocation with associated radial head and coronoid fractures. Isolated fractures that involve the tip of the coronoid do not require fixation if the elbow remains stable. These fractures should not be thought of as simple avulsion fractures, however, based on the fact that there are no soft tissue attachments to the tip of the coronoid seen on arthrotomy, arthroscopy, and an anatomic study [41]. Axial loading that causes shear is the cause for most coronoid fractures [42]. Isolated coronoid fractures are similar morphologically to coronoid fractures seen in elbow fracture dislocations [40].

Fractures that involves more than 50% of the coronoid have been shown to significantly increase varus-valgus laxity, even in the setting of repaired collateral ligaments (Fig. 8) [31,43]. In the setting

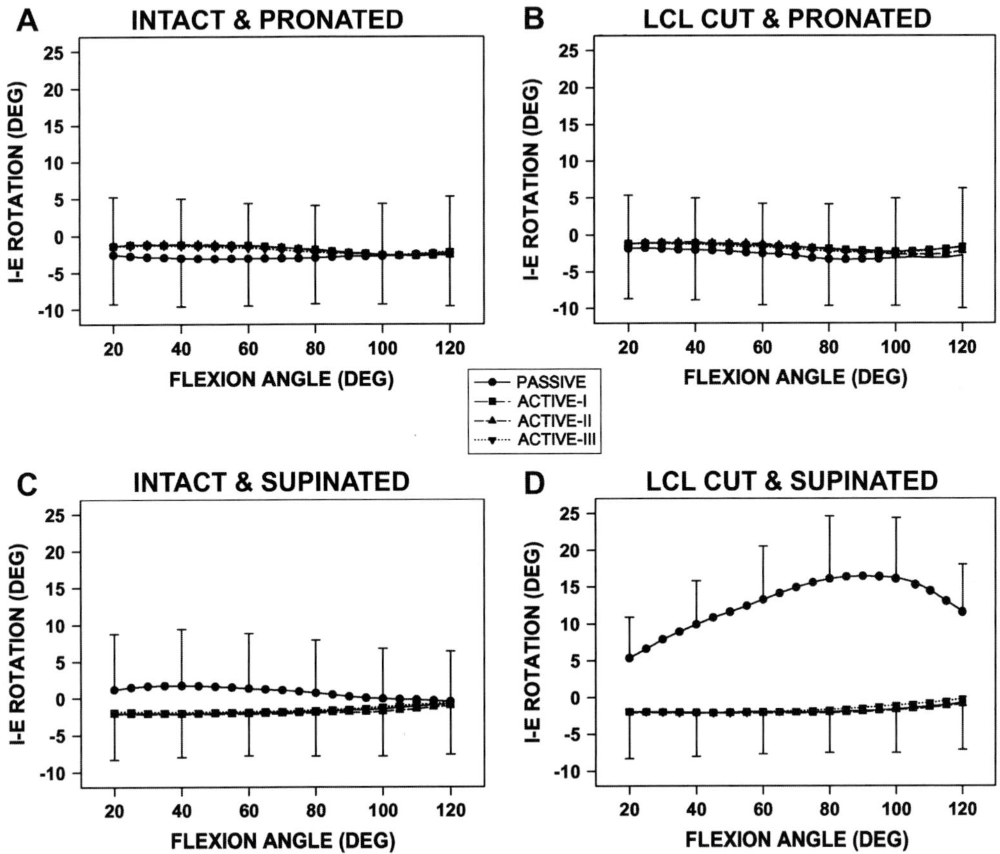

Fig. 7. Mean internal-external (I-E) rotation of the ulna with respect to the humerus is shown for simulated elbow flexion with the forearm in pronation (*A* and *B*) and supination (*C* and *D*) for intact (*A* and *C*) and LCL-deficient (*B* and *D*) elbows (positive = external rotation). Elbow flexion was produced passively and actively. Three different loading combinations (ACTIVE I-III) of the biceps, brachialis, brachioradialis, and triceps were used to generate active flexion. With the forearm pronated, there were no significant differences in I-E rotation between the intact and LCL-deficient elbows with passive or active flexion. With the forearm supinated, however, there was a significant increase in external rotation for passive flexion in the intact and LCL-deficient elbows. The increase in external rotational instability was greatest for the passively flexed LCL-deficient elbow. (*From* Dunning CE, Duck TR, King GJ, et al. Simulated active control produces repeatable motion pathways of the elbow in an in vitro testing system. J Biomech 2001;34(8):1044; with permission.)

of intact ligaments, coronoid fractures that involve more than 50% of the coronoid cause the elbow to became displaced posteriorly more readily than those with less than 50% of the coronoid fractured, especially when the elbow is flexed more than 60° [44]. The coronoid plays a significant role in posterolateral stability in combination with the radial head. With 30% of the coronoid height removed and excision of the radial head, the ulnohumeral joint was shown to dislocate. Stability was restored with replacement of the radial head. With 50% of the coronoid height removed, however, the elbow could not be stabilized with radial head

replacement alone. Subsequent coronoid reconstruction restored stability [45]. Soft tissues that attach to the base of the coronoid include insertion of the anterior capsule and brachialis anteriorly and insertion of the MCL medially. Reduction and fixation of coronoid fractures help to restore the actions of these stabilizers [40].

Olecranon

Treatment of displaced olecranon fractures has been controversial. Excision of the fragment and reattachment of the triceps, especially for elderly patients, became popularized in the 1940s. It was

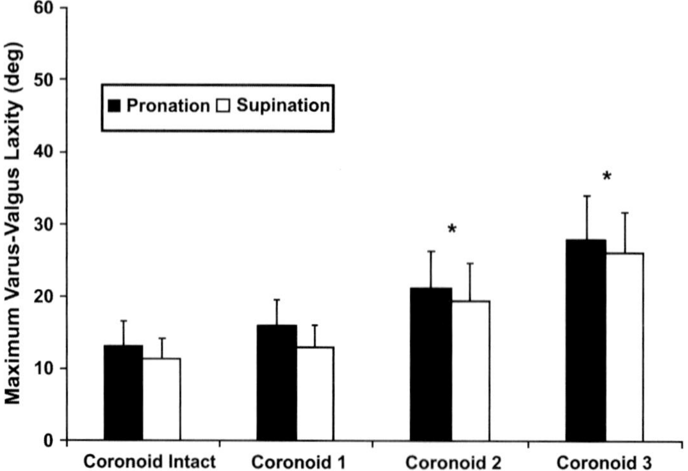

Fig. 8. Average maximum varus-valgus laxity after repair of collateral ligaments with intact coronoid, and simulated coronoid fractures. Coronoid 1 = 10% of bone removed from coronoid tip; coronoid 2 = 50% removed; coronoid 3 = 90% removed. There was significant laxity after 50% of the coronoid was removed. (*From* Beingessner DM, Dunning CE, Stacpoole RA, et al. The effect of coronoid fractures on elbow kinematics and stability. Clin Biomech 2007;22(2):188; with permission.)

stated that as much as 80% of the olecranon could be removed without compromising elbow stability [46]. One study reported that there were no significant differences in elbow extensor power between olecranonectomy with triceps reattachment and open reduction internal fixation of olecranon fractures at an average follow-up time of 3.6 years [47]. In vitro testing of the elbow showed that the constraint of the ulnohumeral joint is linearly proportional to the area of remaining articular surface, from which it was concluded that olecranonectomy is inadvisable in circumstances in which there is instability or an associated coronoid fracture or in a patient with high demands [48]. There are significant increases in joint pressure with excision of 50% of the olecranon, which over time may contribute to elbow pain and arthritis [49].

Proximal radius

The radial head is an important secondary valgus stabilizer of the elbow [36,50,51]. The radial head is responsible for approximately 30% of the valgus stability of the elbow [50]. The radial head becomes more important for valgus stability in the presence of MCL deficiency. When the MCL is transected, replacement of the radial head has been shown to restore valgus stability to a level similar to that of an elbow with an intact radial head [52]. Complete valgus stability is not restored until the MCL is repaired or reconstructed, however [53]. In the presence of an intact MCL, the

radial head may be excised without concern for altering the biomechanics of the elbow [51]. This finding has been challenged more recently by demonstration of posterolateral rotatory instability after isolated excision of the radial head, possibly as a result of decreased tension in the LCL [54]. Radial head excision also increases varus-valgus laxity, regardless of whether the collateral ligaments are intact (Fig. 9) [55].

Soft tissue stabilization

Medial collateral ligament complex

Multiple studies have demonstrated that the AMCL is the primary constraint for valgus and posteromedial stability [11,36,50,51,56,57]. The anterior band of the AMCL is more vulnerable to valgus stress when the elbow is extended, whereas the posterior band is more vulnerable when the elbow is flexed. This finding was supported by an in vitro study, which demonstrated that the anterior band was the primary restraint to valgus stress at 30°, 60°, and 90°, and a coprimary restraint at 120°. The posterior band was a coprimary restraint at 120° and a secondary restraint at 30°, 60°, and 90° [10]. A traumatic valgus force with the elbow flexed at 90° or less is more likely to injure only the anterior band, whereas the elbow flexed more than 90° is more likely to injure the complete AMCL. Complete division of the AMCL causes valgus and internal

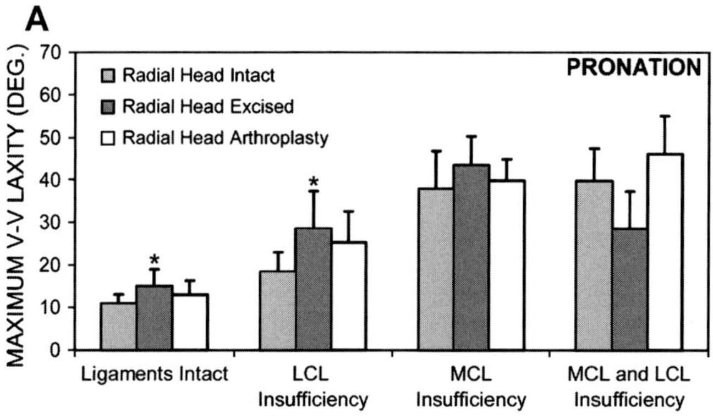

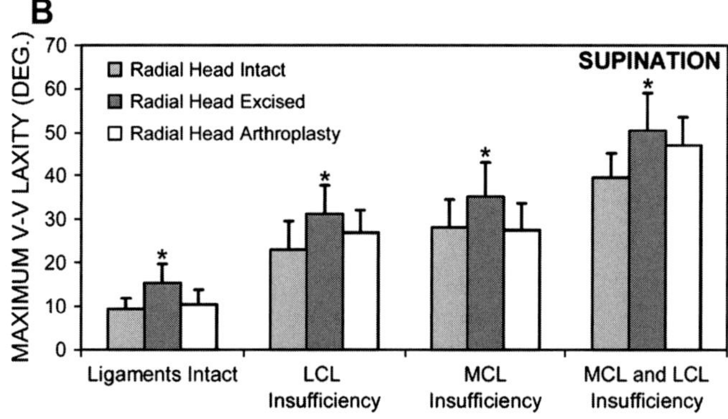

Fig. 9. Maximum varus-valgus laxity plotted for intact and insufficient collateral ligaments with radial head intact, excised, and replaced. Significant increases in laxity after radial head excision are denoted by asterisks. (*From* Beingessner DM, Dunning CE, Gordon KD, et al. The effect of radial head excision and arthroplasty on elbow kinematics and stability. J Bone Joint Surg Am 2004;86(8):1735; with permission.)

rotatory instability throughout the complete arch of flexion with maximal valgus instability at 70° and maximal rotational instability at 60° [11]. The posterior bundle seems to contribute little to valgus stability but does play a role in posteromedial rotatory stability. Severance of the entire posterior band results in only internal rotatory laxity that is maximal at 130° of flexion [11].

The origin of the MCL on the medial epicondyle is posterior to the axis of elbow flexion, which creates a cam-like effect with changes in ligament tension throughout flexion and extension of the elbow. The AMCL increases by 18% from 0° to 120° of flexion [12]. In addition to the anterior and posterior bands of the AMCL, a middle or central band of fibers has been identified that has its proximal origin close to the axis of rotation of the ulnohumeral joint. This central band has been called the "guiding" band because it is nearly isometric and close to being taut throughout the full arc of flexion. When sectioned, there is significant elbow

instability (Fig. 10A) [13,14,58,59]. Single-strand reconstruction of the central band in the MCL-deficient elbow has been shown to restore valgus stability to the elbow similar to the intact condition (Fig. 10B) [60].

LCL complex

The LCL is the primary constraint of external rotation and varus stress at the elbow. The flexion axis of the elbow passes through the origin of the LCL so that there is uniform tension in the ligament throughout the arc of flexion [12]. It has been stated that damage to the LCL complex is the initial injury seen along the continuum of injuries resulting from elbow dislocation [1]. Instability caused by disruption of the LCL must be considered when treating complex fracture dislocations of the elbow. It has been shown that complete sectioning of the LCL causes varus and posterolateral rotatory instability and posterior radial head subluxation [61]. There is disagreement in the literature regarding the exact

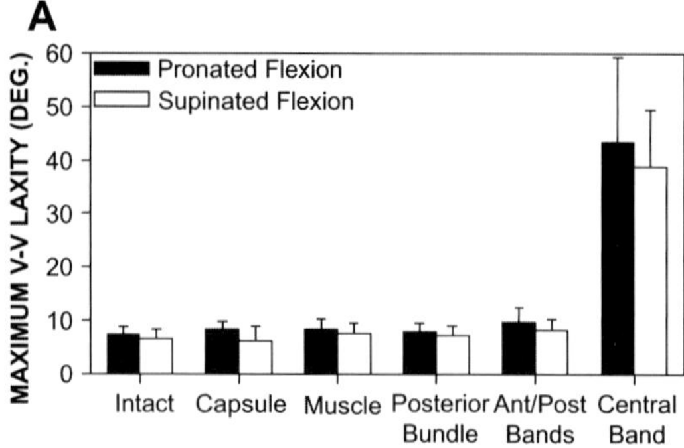

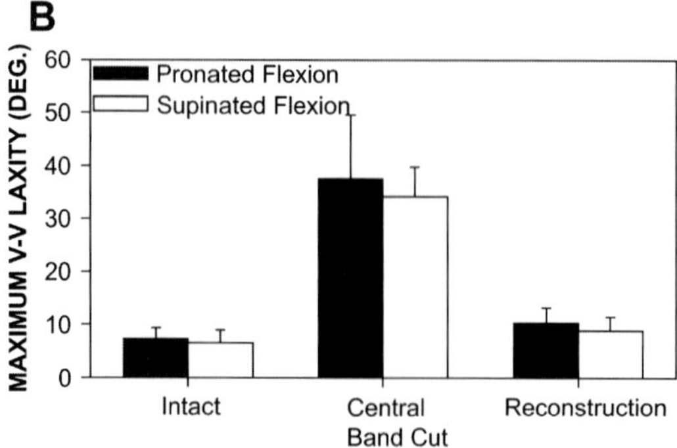

Fig. 10. (*A*) Maximum varus-valgus (V-V) laxity with forearm pronation and supination is plotted for the intact elbow and after sectioning each of the medial elbow stabilizers. The only significant difference in varus-valgus laxity among the structures sectioned occurred after the central band was cut. (*B*) Reconstruction of the central band of the AMCL decreases varus-valgus laxity so that it is not significantly different than the intact elbow. (*From* Armstrong AD, Dunning CE, Faber KJ, et al. Single strand ligament reconstruction of the medial collateral ligament restores valgus elbow stability. J Shoulder Elbow Surg 2002;11(1):69; with permission.)

role of each portion of the LCL complex [62–67]. Recent research has suggested that the LCL complex acts as one functional unit rather than each portion having its own stabilizing function. When the annular ligament and the lateral ulnar collateral ligament are cut in isolation there is only minor laxity [68]. If the annular ligament is intact, the lateral ulnar collateral ligament and radial collateral ligament need to be transected to produce significant posterolateral rotatory and varus-valgus instability (Fig. 11) [63]. This has implications for surgeons who are planning lateral surgical approaches to the elbow for radial head fixation or replacement. As long as the annular ligament is intact, the radial collateral ligament or the lateral ulnar collateral ligament can be cut and repaired without causing instability [63].

When the radial head is excised in the presence of a deficient LCL, there is increased varus and external rotatory instability. Radial head replacement in this setting improves posterolateral instability. Complete stability is not restored until the LCL complex is repaired, however [69]. Although the radial head plays a role in providing stability to the lateral aspect of the elbow, the LCL complex is the primary constraint for varus and external rotatory stability. It is recommended that the LCL complex be repaired after radial head fixation or replacement, particularly in complex elbow fracture dislocation injuries [69].

Muscles

Muscles that cross the elbow joint act as dynamic stabilizers as they compress the joint. Multiple studies have demonstrated the stabilizing effects of loading the muscles that cross the unstable elbow joint [28–30,70,71]. Dynamic compression of the elbow has been shown to decrease the variability of motion pathways of the articulating surfaces at the joint and increases the constraint (Fig. 12) [71].

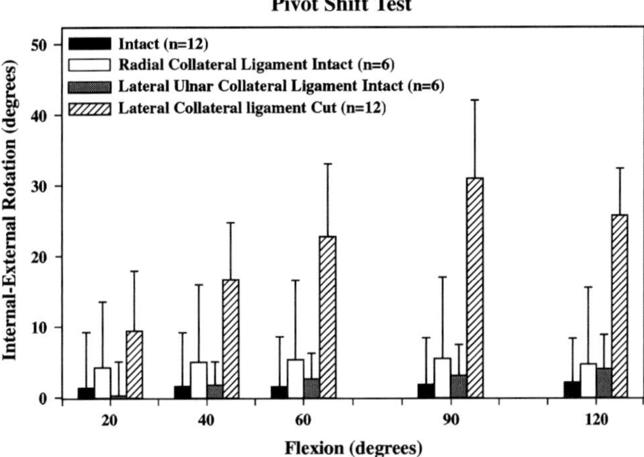

Fig. 11. Mean internal-external elbow rotation during the pivot shift test is plotted for the intact elbow and after sectioning components of lateral collateral ligament. The only significant difference occurred after sectioning of the complete LCL. (*From* Dunning CE, Zarzour ZD, Patterson SD, et al. Ligamentous stabilizers against posterolateral rotatory instability of the elbow. J Bone Joint Surg Am 2001;83(12):1826; with permission.)

Compression of the elbow joint by the muscles protects the soft tissue constraints. For example, throwing an object can cause a valgus stress that is greater than the failure strength of the MCL. The flexor-pronator muscle group contracts during the throwing motion and provides dynamic stabilization to the medial aspect of the elbow, which protects the MCL from injury [72].

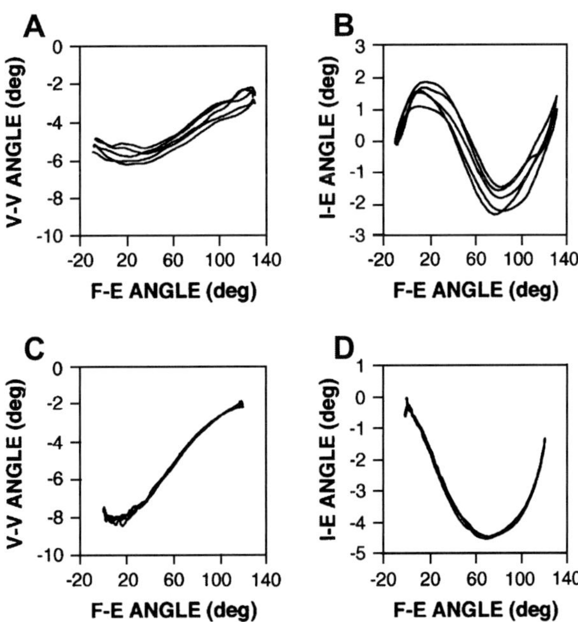

Fig. 12. Motion pathways of the ulna relative to the humerus during repeated flexion of the elbow under passive (*A* and *B*) and active (*C* and *D*) muscle conditions. F-E, flexion-extension; V-V Angle, varus-valgus angulation of elbow during flexion; I-E angle, internal-external rotation of the forearm during elbow flexion. (*From* Johnson JA, Rath DA, Dunning CE, et al. Simulation of elbow and forearm motion in vitro using a load controlled testing apparatus. J Biomech 2000;33(5):637; with permission.)

Joint forces

The compressive and shear forces at the elbow are significant. Given the forces that are generated across the joint under some conditions, some clinicians have said that it is "erroneous to think of the elbow as 'non weightbearing'" [42]. Most elbow dislocations occur during a fall onto an outstretched hand. A fall onto an outstretched hand from a height of only 6 cm is estimated to create an axial joint compression force at the elbow of 50% of body weight [73]. Falls from a standing height would be expected to create a significantly greater force. Performing push-ups, a common exercise, has been shown to create an average force of 45% of body weight across the elbow joint [74].

Loads across the elbow have been shown to be distributed 43% across the ulnohumeral joint and 57% across the radiocapitellar joint [75]. Joint reaction forces vary with elbow position. Force transmission at the radiocapitellar joint is greatest between 0° and 30° of flexion and is greater in pronation than in supination [76]. When the elbow is extended, the overall force on the ulnohumeral joint is more concentrated at the coronoid; as the elbow is flexed, the force moves toward the olecranon (Fig. 13) [77].

Summary

Competent diagnosis and treatment of the injured elbow require a systematic approach and consideration of the anatomy and function of each of the structures that provides stability. Numerous biomechanical studies have contributed greatly to our understanding of elbow motion, forces, and stabilizing factors. Forces across the elbow joint can be significant. Static and dynamic constraints function together to protect the elbow. Each of the three primary constraints must be addressed after elbow trauma for restoration of stability. Secondary constraints, such as the radial head, also play an important role in providing stability. Awareness of the function and likelihood of injury of each stabilizing structure is needed for proficient management of elbow trauma.

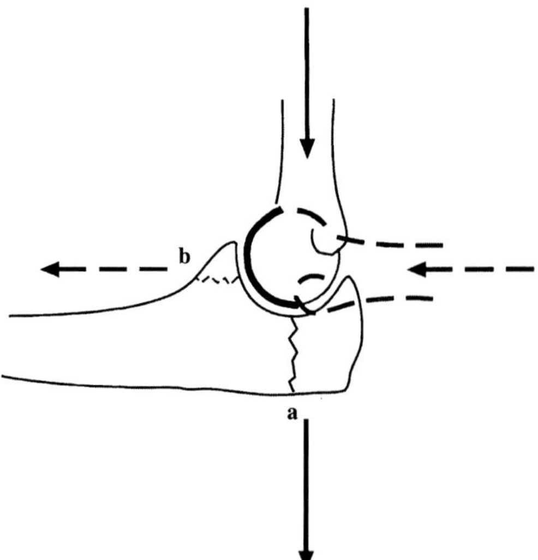

Fig. 13. Concentration of the force at the ulnohumeral joint varies with flexion and extension of the elbow. When the elbow is flexed at 90° (*solid line*), force is concentrated at the olecranon. When the elbow is extended (*dashed line*) the forced is concentrated at the coronoid. The olecranon fracture (a) and coronoid fracture (b) are shown. (*Adapted from* Wake H, Hashizume H, Nishida K, et al. Biomechanical analysis of the mechanism of elbow fracture-dislocations by compression force. J Orthop Sci 2004;9(1):49; with permission.)

References

[1] O'Driscoll SW, Jupiter JB, King GJ, et al. The unstable elbow. Instr Course Lect 2001;50:89–102.

[2] Prasad A, Robertson DD, Sharma GB, et al. Elbow: the trochleogingylomoid joint. Semin Musculoskelet Radiol 2003;7(1):19–25.

[3] Miyasaka KC. Anatomy of the elbow. Orthop Clin North Am 1999;30(1):1–13.

[4] King GJ, Zarzour ZD, Patterson SD, et al. An anthropometric study of the radial head: implications in the design of a prosthesis. J Arthroplasty 2001;16(1):112–6.

[5] Armstrong AD, King GJ, Yamaguchi K. Total elbow arthroplasty design. In: Williams GR, Yamaguchi K, Ramsey ML, et al, editors. Shoulder and elbow arthroplasty. Philadelphia: Lippincott Williams & Wilkins; 2005. p. 297–312.

[6] Johnson JA, King GJ. Anatomy and biomechanics of the elbow. In: Williams GR, Yamaguchi K, Ramsey ML, et al, editors. Shoulder and elbow arthroplasty. Philadelphia: Lippincott Williams and Wilkins; 2005. p. 279–96.

[7] Gallay SH, Richards RR, O'Driscoll SW. Intraarticular capacity and compliance of stiff and normal elbows. Arthroscopy 1993;9(1):9–13.

[8] O'Driscoll SW, Morrey BF, An KN. Intraarticular pressure and capacity of the elbow. Arthroscopy 1990;6(2):100–3.

[9] Deutch SR, Olsen BS, Jensen SL, et al. Ligamentous and capsular restraints to experimental posterior elbow joint dislocation. Scand J Med Sci Sports 2003;13(5):311–6.

[10] Callaway GH, Field LD, Deng XH, et al. Biomechanical evaluation of the medial collateral ligament of the elbow. J Bone Joint Surg Am 1997;79(8):1223–31.

[11] Floris S, Olsen BS, Dalstra M, et al. The medial collateral ligament of the elbow joint: anatomy and kinematics. J Shoulder Elbow Surg 1998;7(4): 345–51.

[12] Morrey BF, An KN. Functional anatomy of the ligaments of the elbow. Clin Orthop Relat Res 1985; 201:84–90.

[13] Fuss FK. The ulnar collateral ligament of the human elbow joint: anatomy, function and biomechanics. J Anat 1991;175:203–12.

[14] Ochi N, Ogura T, Hashizume H, et al. Anatomic relation between the medial collateral ligament of the elbow and the humero-ulnar joint axis. J Shoulder Elbow Surg 1999;8(1):6–10.

[15] O'Driscoll SW, Bell DF, Morrey BF. Posterolateral rotatory instability of the elbow. J Bone Joint Surg Am 1991;73(3):440–6.

[16] Boone DC, Azen SP. Normal range of motion of joints in male subjects. J Bone Joint Surg Am 1979; 61(5):756–9.

[17] Morrey BF, Askew LJ, Chao EY. A biomechanical study of normal functional elbow motion. J Bone Joint Surg Am 1981;63(6):872–7.

[18] Morrey BF, Chao EY. Passive motion of the elbow joint. J Bone Joint Surg Am 1976;58(4):501–8.

[19] Bottlang M, Madey SM, Steyers CM, et al. Assessment of elbow joint kinematics in passive motion by electromagnetic motion tracking. J Orthop Res 2000;18(2):195–202.

[20] Duck TR, Dunning CE, King GJ, et al. Variability and repeatability of the flexion axis at the ulnohumeral joint. J Orthop Res 2003;21(3):399–404.

[21] Ericson A, Arndt A, Stark A, et al. Variation in the position and orientation of the elbow flexion axis. J Bone Joint Surg Br 2003;85(4):538–44.

[22] Stokdijk M, Meskers CG, Veeger HE, et al. Determination of the optimal elbow axis for evaluation of placement of prostheses. Clin Biomech (Bristol, Avon) 1999;14(3):177–84.

[23] Brownhill JR, Furukawa K, Faber KJ, et al. Surgeon accuracy in the selection of the flexion-extension axis of the elbow: an in vitro study. J Shoulder Elbow Surg 2006;15(4):451–6.

[24] Kapandji A. Biomechanics of pronation and supination of the forearm. Hand Clin 2001;17(1):111–22.

[25] Hollister AM, Gellman H, Waters RL. The relationship of the interosseous membrane to the axis of rotation of the forearm. Clin Orthop Relat Res 1994;298:272–6.

[26] Moore DC, Hogan KA, Crisco JJ III, et al. Three-dimensional in vivo kinematics of the distal radioulnar joint in malunited distal radius fractures. J Hand Surg [Am] 2002;27(2):233–42.

[27] Palmer AK, Werner FW. Biomechanics of the distal radioulnar joint. Clin Orthop Relat Res 1984;187: 26–35.

[28] Dunning CE, Zarzour ZD, Patterson SD, et al. Muscle forces and pronation stabilize the lateral ligament deficient elbow. Clin Orthop Relat Res 2001;388:118–24.

[29] Armstrong AD, Dunning CE, Faber KJ, et al. Rehabilitation of the medial collateral ligament-deficient elbow: an in vitro biomechanical study. J Hand Surg [Am] 2000;25(6):1051–7.

[30] Dunning CE, Duck TR, King GJ, et al. Simulated active control produces repeatable motion pathways of the elbow in an in vitro testing system. J Biomech 2001;34(8):1039–48.

[31] Beingessner DM, Dunning CE, Stacpoole RA, et al. The effect of coronoid fractures on elbow kinematics and stability. Clin Biomech (Bristol, Avon) 2007; 22(2):183–90.

[32] Safran MR, McGarry MH, Shin S, et al. Effects of elbow flexion and forearm rotation on valgus laxity of the elbow. J Bone Joint Surg Am 2005;87(9): 2065–74.

[33] Eygendaal D, Verdegaal SH, Obermann WR, et al. Posterolateral dislocation of the elbow joint: relationship to medial instability. J Bone Joint Surg Am 2000; 82(4):555–60.

[34] Josefsson PO, Gentz CF, Johnell O, et al. Surgical versus non-surgical treatment of ligamentous injuries following dislocation of the elbow joint: a prospective randomized study. J Bone Joint Surg Am 1987;69(4):605–8.

[35] Josefsson PO, Johnell O, Wendeberg B. Ligamentous injuries in dislocations of the elbow joint. Clin Orthop Relat Res 1987;221:221–5.

[36] Morrey BF, An KN. Articular and ligamentous contributions to the stability of the elbow joint. Am J Sports Med 1983;11(5):315–9.

[37] Josefsson PO, Gentz CF, Johnell O, et al. Dislocations of the elbow and intraarticular fractures. Clin Orthop Relat Res 1989;246:126–30.

[38] Morrey BF. Complex instability of the elbow. Instr Course Lect 1998;47:157–64.

[39] Regan W, Morrey BF. Classification and treatment of coronoid process fractures. Orthopedics 1992; 15(7):845–8.

[40] McKee MD, Jupiter JB. Trauma of the adult elbow and fractures of the distal humerus. In: Browner BD, Jupiter JB, Levine AM, et al, editors. 3rd edition. Skeletal trauma: basic science, management, and reconstruction, vol. 2. Philadelphia: Saunders; 2003. p. 1404–80.

[41] Cage DJ, Abrams RA, Callahan JJ, et al. Soft tissue attachments of the ulnar coronoid process: an anatomic study with radiographic correlation. Clin Orthop Relat Res 1995;320:154–8.

[42] Amis AA, Dowson D, Wright V. Elbow joint force predictions for some strenuous isometric actions. J Biomech 1980;13(9):765–75.

[43] Hull JR, Owen JR, Fern SE, et al. Role of the coronoid process in varus osteoarticular stability of the elbow. J Shoulder Elbow Surg 2005;14(4):441–6.

[44] Closkey RF, Goode JR, Kirschenbaum D, et al. The role of the coronoid process in elbow stability: a biomechanical analysis of axial loading. J Bone Joint Surg Am 2000;82(12):1749–53.

[45] Schneeberger AG, Sadowski MM, Jacob HA. Coronoid process and radial head as posterolateral rotatory stabilizers of the elbow. J Bone Joint Surg Am 2004;86(5):975–82.

[46] McKeever F, Buck R. Fracture of the olecranon process of the ulna. JAMA 1947;135(1):1–5.

[47] Gartsman GM, Sculco TP, Otis JC. Operative treatment of olecranon fractures: excision or open reduction with internal fixation. J Bone Joint Surg Am 1981;63(5):718–21.

[48] An KN, Morrey BF, Chao EY. The effect of partial removal of proximal ulna on elbow constraint. Clin Orthop Relat Res 1986;209:270–9.

[49] Moed BR, Ede DE, Brown TD. Fractures of the olecranon: an in vitro study of elbow joint stresses after tension-band wire fixation versus proximal fracture fragment excision. J Trauma 2002;53(6):1088–93.

[50] Hotchkiss RN, Weiland AJ. Valgus stability of the elbow. J Orthop Res 1987;5(3):372–7.

[51] Morrey BF, Tanaka S, An KN. Valgus stability of the elbow: a definition of primary and secondary constraints. Clin Orthop Relat Res 1991;265:187–95.

[52] Johnson JA, Beingessner DM, Gordon KD, et al. Kinematics and stability of the fractured and implant-reconstructed radial head. J Shoulder Elbow Surg 2005;14(1 Suppl S):195S–201S.

[53] King GJ, Zarzour ZD, Rath DA, et al. Metallic radial head arthroplasty improves valgus stability of the elbow. Clin Orthop Relat Res 1999;368:114–25.

[54] Sojbjerg JO, Ovesen J, Gundorf CE. The stability of the elbow following excision of the radial head and transection of the annular ligament: an experimental study. Arch Orthop Trauma Surg 1987;106(4):248–50.

[55] Beingessner DM, Dunning CE, Gordon KD, et al. The effect of radial head excision and arthroplasty on elbow kinematics and stability. J Bone Joint Surg Am 2004;86(8):1730–9.

[56] Schwab GH, Bennett JB, Woods GW, et al. Biomechanics of elbow instability: the role of the medial collateral ligament. Clin Orthop Relat Res 1980;146:42–52.

[57] Sojbjerg JO, Ovesen J, Nielsen S. Experimental elbow instability after transection of the medial collateral ligament. Clin Orthop Relat Res 1987;218:186–90.

[58] Armstrong AD, Ferreira LM, Dunning CE, et al. The medial collateral ligament of the elbow is not isometric: an in vitro biomechanical study. Am J Sports Med 2004;32(1):85–90.

[59] Regan WD, Korinek SL, Morrey BF, et al. Biomechanical study of ligaments around the elbow joint. Clin Orthop Relat Res 1991;271:170–9.

[60] Armstrong AD, Dunning CE, Faber KJ, et al. Single strand ligament reconstruction of the medial collateral ligament restores valgus elbow stability. J Shoulder Elbow Surg 2002;11(1):65–77.

[61] Olsen BS, Vaesel MT, Sojbjerg JO, et al. Lateral collateral ligament of the elbow joint: anatomy and kinematics. J Shoulder Elbow Surg 1996;5(2 Pt 1):103–12.

[62] Cohen MS, Hastings H II. Rotatory instability of the elbow: the anatomy and role of the lateral stabilizers. J Bone Joint Surg Am 1997;79(2):225–33.

[63] Dunning CE, Zarzour ZD, Patterson SD, et al. Ligamentous stabilizers against posterolateral rotatory instability of the elbow. J Bone Joint Surg Am 2001;83(12):1823–8.

[64] Imatani J, Ogura T, Morito Y, et al. Anatomic and histologic studies of lateral collateral ligament complex of the elbow joint. J Shoulder Elbow Surg 1999;8(6):625–7.

[65] McAdams TR, Masters GW, Srivastava S. The effect of arthroscopic sectioning of the lateral ligament complex of the elbow on posterolateral rotatory stability. J Shoulder Elbow Surg 2005;14(3):298–301.

[66] Olsen BS, Sojbjerg JO, Nielsen KK, et al. Posterolateral elbow joint instability: the basic kinematics. J Shoulder Elbow Surg 1998;7(1):19–29.

[67] Seki A, Olsen BS, Jensen SL, et al. Functional anatomy of the lateral collateral ligament complex of the elbow: configuration of Y and its role. J Shoulder Elbow Surg 2002;11(1):53–9.

[68] Olsen BS, Sojbjerg JO, Dalstra M, et al. Kinematics of the lateral ligamentous constraints of the elbow joint. J Shoulder Elbow Surg 1996;5(5):333–41.

[69] Jensen SL, Olsen BS, Tyrdal S, et al. Elbow joint laxity after experimental radial head excision and lateral collateral ligament rupture: efficacy of prosthetic replacement and ligament repair. J Shoulder Elbow Surg 2005;14(1):78–84.

[70] Buchanan TS, Delp SL, Solbeck JA. Muscular resistance to varus and valgus loads at the elbow. J Biomech Eng 1998;120(5):634–9.

[71] Johnson JA, Rath DA, Dunning CE, et al. Simulation of elbow and forearm motion in vitro using a load controlled testing apparatus. J Biomech 2000;33(5):635–9.

[72] Park MC, Ahmad CS. Dynamic contributions of the flexor-pronator mass to elbow valgus stability. J Bone Joint Surg Am 2004;86(10):2268–74.

[73] Chou PH, Chou YL, Lin CJ, et al. Effect of elbow flexion on upper extremity impact forces during a fall. Clin Biomech (Bristol, Avon) 2001;16(10):888–94.

[74] An KN, Chao EY, Morrey BF, et al. Intersegmental elbow joint load during pushup. Biomed Sci Instrum 1992;28:69–74.

[75] Halls AA, Travill A. Transmission of pressures across the elbow joint. Anat Rec 1964;150:243–7.

[76] Morrey BF, An KN, Stormont TJ. Force transmission through the radial head. J Bone Joint Surg Am 1988;70(2):250–6.

[77] Wake H, Hashizume H, Nishida K, et al. Biomechanical analysis of the mechanism of elbow fracture-dislocations by compression force. J Orthop Sci 2004;9(1):44–50.

Orthop Clin N Am 39 (2008) 155–161

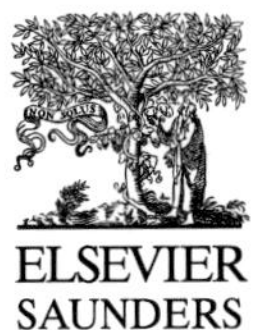

ORTHOPEDIC
CLINICS
OF NORTH AMERICA

Acute Elbow Dislocations

Michael A. Kuhn, MD[a],*, Glen Ross, MD[b]

[a]*Naval Hospital Camp Lejeune, Department of Orthopaedics, 100 Brewster Boulevard, Camp Lejeune, NC 28547, USA*
[b]*Department of Orthopaedics and Sports Medicine, Orthopaedic Sports Medicine, New England Baptist Hospital,
125 Parker Hill Avenue, Boston, MA 02120, USA*

The elbow is the second most commonly dislocated major joint in the adult age group, and the most commonly dislocated major joint in the pediatric population. The incidence of elbow dislocation is 6 of every 100,000 individuals during their lifetime [1]. The nondominant extremity is involved with a slight predominance. It has been suggested that there is a protective instinct using the dominant side to shield from a fall. Elbow dislocations constitute 10% to 25% of all injuries to the elbow. The mean age of an individual sustaining this injury is 30 years. There is a male predominance with 2 to 2.5 times that of females, with similar ratios seen in children. Approximately 40% of elbow dislocations occur during sports. Gymnastics, wrestling, basketball, and football are commonly involved. Approximately 40% of dislocations have a poorly defined mechanism of injury [2].

Etiology

The mechanism of elbow dislocation has been extensively studied through video observation and clinical research. Traditionally, the mechanism of injury was believed to be a hyperextension moment. A fall on the outstretched hand is a common event. The elbow experiences an axial compressive force during flexion as the body approaches the ground. The body rotates internally, with the forearm rotating externally to the trunk, resulting

in a supination moment at the elbow. At that point, the mechanical axis of the extremity is medial to the elbow resulting in a valgus moment. O'Driscoll and Morrey [3] suggested that an extension varus stress disrupts the lateral ligament complex first. A perched dislocation results if the force of the fall is dissipated at this moment. If the disruptive force continues, forearm rotation occurs, resulting in the tearing of the capsule and finally a complete dislocation. The final disruption occurs to the medial structures. This disruption has been described as the "ring of instability" progressing from disruption of the lateral ulnar collateral ligament, to the capsule, and finally injury to the medial ulnar collateral ligament. With a slightly flexed elbow, a tear in the medial collateral ligament complex occurs and the elbow dislocates [2].

The disruptive forces around the ligamentous structures of the elbow also include substantial compressive and shear forces occurring on the articular surfaces. Dissipation of this force can cause fractures of the proximal radius and significant cartilaginous injuries. Dislocations treated by open procedures have documented chondral injuries to the capitellum and trochlear surfaces at higher rates than previously believed. Understanding the mechanism of injury is important for appreciating classification, interpreting radiographs, formulating a treatment plan, anticipating complications, and guiding follow-up care.

* Corresponding author. Department of Orthopaedics, Orthopaedic Sports Medicine, Camp Lejeune Naval Hospital, 100 Brewster Blvd., Camp Lejeune, NC 28547.
   E-mail address: drmakuhn@hotmail.com (M.A. Kuhn).

Pathophysiology

O'Driscoll's [2] ring of instability has been broken into stages of disruption and a classification of elbow dislocations. Stage 1 involves disruption

0030-5898/08/$ - see front matter © 2008 Elsevier Inc. All rights reserved.
doi:10.1016/j.ocl.2007.12.004

of the ulnar component of the lateral collateral ligament. Posterolateral rotatory subluxation of the elbow results and the elbow reduces spontaneously. With continued force, disruption occurs anteriorly and posteriorly allowing for an incomplete posterolateral dislocation, which has been described as a perched dislocation. Stage 3 has been subdivided into two parts. In stage 3A, all soft tissues are disrupted around to and including the posterior part of the medial collateral ligament. The anterior band of the medial collateral ligament remains intact, allowing for posterior dislocation by the previously described posterolateral rotatory mechanism. In stage 3B, the entire medial collateral complex is disrupted. Varus, valgus, and rotatory instability are present. Surgical experience suggests that the medial collateral complex is disrupted in nearly 100% of elbow dislocations. Violation of the anterior bundle of the medial collateral ligament is considered the essential lesion. Disruption of this bundle most commonly occurs from the humeral origin.

Dislocation is the final of three sequential stages of elbow instability, resulting from posterolateral ulnohumeral rotatory subluxation, with soft tissue disruption occurring from lateral to medial.

Classification

Elbow dislocations have been traditionally described by the resulting location of the injury. This classification divides elbow dislocations into posterior, anterior, and divergent [3,4]. Posterior dislocations are subdivided based on the final relationship between the humerus and olecranon. These include posterior, posterolateral, posteromedial, and pure lateral dislocations. Posterolateral is the most common dislocation, followed by lateral, and least commonly posteromedial. A divergent dislocation is a rare injury, and generally is associated with high-energy trauma. Displacement of the radius from the ulna occurs resulting in disruption of the interosseous membrane, annular ligament, and distal radioulnar joint capsule [5]. Anterior dislocations are uncommon, occurring in only 1% to 2% of elbow dislocations. Anterior dislocations are usually seen in younger individuals.

Morrey proposed a simple classification distinguishing between a perched and complete dislocation [2]. A medial or lateral resting position of the complete dislocation makes little difference with regard to treatment or prognosis. A perched dislocation is one in which the elbow is actually subluxed but the coronoid appears to impinge

on the trochlea. In this type, the ligaments are less severely injured, and rehabilitation can be more rapid and recovery more complete.

Diagnosis

Before any reduction maneuvers, assessment of neurovascular status is mandatory. Postreduction neurovascular changes can result from entrapment of neurovascular structures, and may require emergent surgical intervention. Anteroposterior and lateral radiographs should be obtained if possible. If the dislocation occurs on the field in the presence of a trained physician, immediate reduction maneuvers are often performed before radiographic procedures. Evaluation of associated injuries should be reserved until reduction has been obtained. Computerized tomography and magnetic resonance imaging are often of limited value before reduction maneuvers [1]. These are reserved for use if adequate radiographs cannot be obtained and can be used for later reconstructive planning.

Associated injuries

Associated injuries with elbow dislocation are common [6]. They may result in significant morbidity. Radial head and neck fractures occur in 5% to 10% of elbow dislocations. Avulsion fractures of the medial or the lateral epicondyles occur in approximately 12% of the cases, and coronoid fractures occur in 10% of dislocations. The incidence of associated fractures in children is high, approaching 50% [1]. With open physes, a medial epicondyle avulsion is the most common associated injury. Incarceration of the fragment into the elbow joint can occur. Although pre- and postreduction radiographs reveal periarticular fractures in 12% to 60% of dislocations, operative findings have revealed unrecognized osteochondral injuries in nearly 100% of acute elbow dislocations [7]. The vast majority of these injuries are small fractures not requiring operative intervention.

Neurovascular injuries are rare, but can be potentially devastating. There are multiple case reports of brachial artery injuries with posterior dislocation. Although it may not be necessary to explore the brachial artery routinely if a radial pulse is present, it is accepted that disruption of the brachial artery should be treated with ligation and vein grafting. Median nerve entrapment has been reported with relocation of a dislocated elbow [1,2,6]. The median nerve may be displaced posteriorly through a space created by avulsion of the medial epicondyle or the common flexor origin, which can result in a tension of the median nerve across the margin of the epicondylar flare and may "notch" the bone, producing a late radiographic sign known as Matev sign [8].

After dislocation, extensive soft tissue swelling commonly occurs. Intact structures, including the forearm fascia, the biceps tendon, and the lacertus fibrosis, may exert a constricting effect resulting in increased compartment pressures. Compartment syndrome is possible and should be considered. Careful observation is required and must be differentiated from neurologic stretch injuries.

Treatment

An expeditious atraumatic reduction is the goal. Often the least traumatic reduction can be performed moments after the injury before the onset of muscle spasm and swelling. As previously stated, this should only be attempted with a dislocation that occurs in the presence of a trained medical professional. When an immediate reduction is not possible, reduction is often best accomplished with conscious sedation or general anesthesia with adequate muscle relaxation. Muscle relaxation is the key to joint reduction. Care is taken to avoid multiple reduction attempts, which would increase the risk for chondral injuries.

A prone traction and countertraction maneuver is often successful (Fig. 1) [9]. Reduction is usually achieved by extending the elbow with

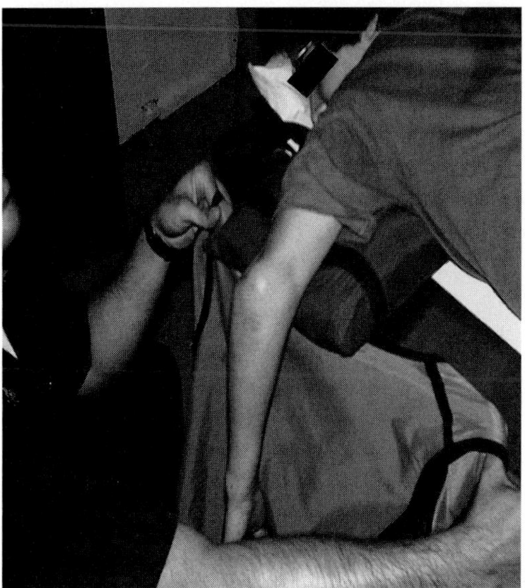

Fig. 1. Prone position for traction countertraction elbow relocation.

countertraction on the arm, and a thumb is used to manipulate the coronoid, clearing the trochlea. Perched dislocation can be treated with intra-articular analgesia and sedation, whereas a complete dislocation may require general anesthesia and a muscle relaxant. Uncommonly, a dislocation occurs that is irreducible by closed reduction. This type of dislocation is most frequently associated with fractures. When a dislocation is irreducible, the radial head has been shown to be trapped in the soft tissues of the forearm or may be interposed through the forearm fascia. These dislocations require surgical intervention. Surgical repair of ligaments without associated fractures in the acute dislocation has not been shown to improve return to activity or function [7].

Following reduction, instability is best assessed with the patient under anesthesia, or with an anesthetized elbow. The quality of joint reduction provides a clue to postreduction stability. Palpating a reduction "clunk" is a favorable sign of joint stability. The elbow is examined for valgus, varus, and posterolateral rotatory instability. Varus and valgus instability are performed with the elbow in full extension and flexion up to 30 degrees. Most dislocated elbows are unstable to a valgus stress. This instability is best tested with the forearm in pronation to lock the lateral side. It is important to evaluate the tendency for redislocation occurring in extension, which can signify a potentially unstable joint. Posterolateral rotatory instability is diagnosed by the lateral pivot-shift test. A positive test is manifested by a clunk that is heard and felt when the ulna and radius reduce on the humerus [1,2].

Postreduction radiographs should be obtained to confirm a concentric reduction. Anteroposterior and lateral views should be obtained. Widening of the joint space may indicate entrapped osteochondral fragments, which must be removed surgically. Posterolateral rotatory instability may also present as a non-concentric reduction.

The wrist and shoulder should be examined to rule out concomitant injuries, which occur in 10% to 15% of cases. The distal radioulnar joint and interosseous membrane should be evaluated for tenderness and instability to rule out injury.

Surgical treatment

All complete elbow dislocations without large periarticular fractures result in medial and lateral ligament ruptures. Rarely is surgical treatment necessary in the acute setting. Josefsson and associates [7] evaluated 31 acute elbow dislocations without concomitant fractures. Under anesthesia 9 were unstable in full extension. They surgically explored all 31 elbows finding ruptures of the medial and lateral ligaments. The tendency of elbows to dislocate correlated with the degree of muscular injury to the flexor-pronator and extensor origins on the humerus. They concluded that muscular flexor and extensor origins represent secondary stabilizers of the elbow. If they are intact, they provide adequate stability to allow ligamentous healing after elbow dislocation. Prospective studies have failed to show improvement of early collateral ligament repair over early motion after a simple elbow dislocation.

Acute surgical intervention is indicated in few incidences. Open elbow dislocation and acute compartment syndrome require urgent intervention. Postreduction instability requiring 50 to 60 degrees of flexion to remain stable may require intervention. Elbow dislocations with unstable fractures require surgical stabilization. The unstable elbow will redislocate even with a well-fitting cast or splint (Fig. 2A–C). If this occurs,

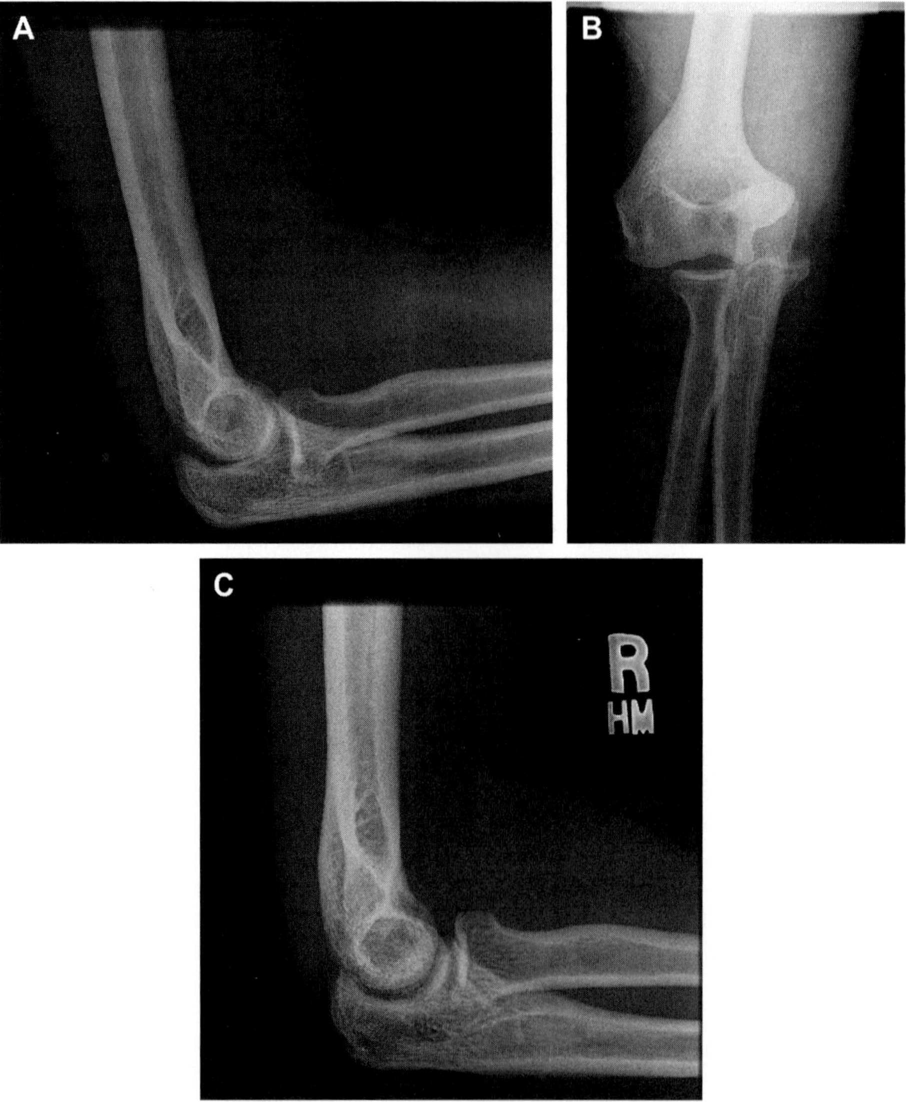

Fig. 2. Patient who had recurrent instability and dislocated 2 weeks after closed reduction. (*A*) The redislocation was not initially recognized with only a lateral radiograph. The joint is not congruent. (*B*) Orthogonal anteroposterior view shows the clear dislocation. (*C*) Lateral radiograph obtained after open repair of medial and lateral ligaments with a congruent, stable joint.

rigid external fixation with pins in the humerus and ulna are required to maintain a stable concentric reduction. Dynamic external fixation may be used allowing motion in the stable range of motion.

Rehabilitation

The results of treatment of a simple closed elbow dislocation are not universally successful. Most authors recommend a period of immobilization lasting from 3 to 10 days [1,2]. Restoration of full range of motion, especially extension, is not reliably achieved. Non-immobilization and early rapid motion under supervision have been shown to achieve range of motion within 5 degrees of extension of the contralateral elbow with an excellent functional outcome. Patients who have persistent loss of motion by 6 to 8 weeks postinjury require additional intervention [1,2,7]. Patient-adjusted static flexion and extension splints are used to facilitate regaining motion. Rehabilitation should be closely supervised, often requiring multiple therapy sessions per week in the acute phase of rehabilitation.

Results

Melhoff and associates [6] reported on the long-term sequelae of simple elbow dislocations. They found a direct correlation with the period of immobilization. Immobilization greater than 3 weeks resulted in a high incidence of contractures. Sixty-five percent reported loss of motion, especially in extension. Uncomplicated dislocations generally have satisfactory results. Excellent results with full range of motion, normal strength, absent pain, and good stability may be expected in 50% of patients. Good results, defined as less than 15 degrees of motion loss, minimal discomfort, and normal stability, may be expected in one third of patients. Fair or poor results are generally associated with complications and severe injuries and occur in 15 % of cases.

Most patients note continued improvement up to 6 months, and rarely up to 18 months [1,2,7,9]. Limitations in extension are the most common problem. Recurrent instability has not been commonly reported, but symptoms have been noted in up to 35 % of cases. Even long after healing, approximately 50% of patients followed up long term complain of discomfort or residual symptoms attributed to their elbow after a dislocation, predominately during heavy loading of the affected extremity. Approximately 60% of patients reported that their elbow did not feel as "good" as the contralateral elbow. Mechanical testing reveals a 15% average loss of elbow strength.

Complications

Posttraumatic stiffness is much more common than instability after elbow dislocation. Limitation of extension is common with frequent loss of 10 to 15 degrees of terminal extension [1,2,7]. Bracing and therapy are not generally useful after 1 year. If there is sufficient limitation of 30 degrees or more, capsulolysis may be considered. The anterior capsule can be released by way of an open or arthroscopic approach.

Heterotopic bone formation occurs at three primary locations following dislocations. Ossification in the lateral and medial collateral ligaments occurs most frequently (reported in approximately 75% of cases), but seldom causes impairment. Ossification occurs in the anterior capsule above the coronoid process. True ectopic ossification that limits motion is rare, occurring in fewer than 5% of cases. Motion-limiting ossification excision is delayed until reactive bone has matured, generally at 1 year.

Neurologic problems occur in up to 20% of dislocations. Symptoms range from transient paresthesia to a rare permanent ulnar palsy. Median nerve involvement is less common. Stretching and distortion of the anterior structures may result in spasm, intimal damage, thrombosis, or rupture of the brachial artery. Because dislocation involves disruption of collateral circulation, the forearm can be placed at risk. Ischemic myositis, myonecrosis, impaired vascularity, or claudication may result.

Compartment syndrome can result from intramuscular bleeding and edema formation within the flexor compartment of the forearm. Pain with passive finger and wrist extension out of proportion to the injury raises clinical suspicion. Compartment pressures are obtained when the diagnosis is in doubt, and arteriography is obtained if arterial injury is suspected.

Elbow dislocations with radial head fractures can be associated with distal radioulnar instability, a variant of the Essex-Lopresti injury. The combined injury makes radial head reconstruction important for elbow stability and axial stability of the forearm. If the radial head is not reconstructible, a metal prosthesis, or allograft radial head, can provide axial support to the radius and improve valgus stability of the elbow. Temporary pin fixation of the distal radioulnar joint in a neutral position may be added to resist the tendency of proximal radial migration.

Authors' preferred treatment

Diagnosis of acute elbow dislocation is usually straightforward, and careful evaluation of radiographs should allow classification of a complex or simple dislocation. Most injuries are simple, without significant associated fracture. A rapid but complete neurovascular assessment is documented.

Reduction is performed expeditiously. On-field reduction may be performed under select conditions if there is an obvious dislocation and an experienced provider at the injury site. Most patients require transportation to an acute care facility for radiographic evaluation.

Ease of reduction is generally inversely proportional to the degree of muscle spasm present. Analgesia may be provided with conscious monitored sedation or regional or general anesthesia. The prone position with an assistant controlling the proximal humerus for traction–countertraction has been helpful. The forearm is supinated, and with pressure on the proximal olecranon, a successful reduction can usually be achieved. The stability of the reduction is assessed with range of motion, and the patient is temporarily placed in a sling for postreduction radiographs.

Most reductions are stable. We have found for this group an aggressive early ROM protocol emphasizing active motion has been helpful for maximizing final range of motion and minimizing extension loss (Table 1) [9]. Rarely, an elbow dislocation without fracture will be grossly unstable following reduction. In this circumstance, an early MRI, followed by exploration and repair of the medial collateral ligament, flexor-pronator tendon, and lateral ulnar collateral ligament can restore stability. Dynamic external fixation is another option. Our experience has been that early

Table 1
Elbow dislocation protocol

Daily measurements	Before treatment: (1) Measure arm circumference 3 in above and 3 in below the medial epicondyle; (2) measure elbow range of motion. After treatment: Measure elbow range of motion
Treatment day 1	Begin with neuromuscular electrical stimulation under cold water for 20 min. Immediately after the treatment, place the athlete supine on a table. Use a 6-in latex compression wrap to apply compression from distal to proximal (metacarpophalangeal joints to the top of the shoulder). The injured extremity should be elevated above the heart. Maintain compression for 60 s on, then 60 s off, for a total treatment time of 30 min. Unwrap the bandage rapidly (the patient will feel the blood rush to the hand). On release of the wrap, instruct the athlete to open and close the hand rapidly while simultaneously working on flexion and extension of the elbow. This must be a pain-free active (not passive) exercise. After treatment, use a doubled 3-in rubberized stockinette from the metacarpophalangeal joints to the top of the shoulder to secure two 5-in oval foam pads to the elbow. Place the pads over the condyles, with the sleeve maintaining their position to provide gentle compression. The sleeve should be removed only for treatment. The entire procedure should be comfortable for the patient.
Treatment day 2	Repeat day 1 modalities. Replace the pads and sleeve. Also, instruct the patient to do a bounce/catch/squeeze exercise using a tennis ball, incorporating biceps flexion/extension, and wrist pronation/supination through a pain-free range of motion. This exercise can be accomplished during short, intermittent breaks throughout the day.
Treatment days 3 and 4	Repeat day 1 modalities. On completion, instruct the patient in using the injured extremity in the swimming pool. Breast stroke for 30 to 45 min is recommended. If available, begin use of an Upper Body Exerciser (UBE, Cybex, Ronkonkoma, New York). Adjust the UBE handgrip length to accommodate for the injury and the tolerable range of elbow motion. After exercise, ice the elbow for 20 min, and replace the pads and sleeves for compression.
Treatment days 5–7	Repeat day 1 modalities. Continue with the compression wrap routine until swelling is reduced to within 1 cm of the contralateral elbow. At that time, begin isokinetic exercises, focusing on wrist flexion/extension/pronation/supination, and biceps/triceps strengthening. After exercise, ice the elbow for 20 min and replace the pads and sleeve for elbow compression until edema is completely eliminated.

range of motion is critical to ensuring a successful outcome.

Summary

Diagnosis of acute elbow dislocation is usually straightforward, and careful evaluation of radiographs should allow classification of a complex or simple dislocation. Assessment of neurovascular status is mandatory before reduction maneuvers. Posttraumatic stiffness is much more common than instability after elbow dislocation. For stable elbow dislocations, an aggressive early ROM protocol emphasizing active motion has been helpful for maximizing final range of motion, minimizing extension loss, improving patient satisfaction, and improving ultimate outcomes.

References

[1] Mezera K, Hotchkiss RN. Fractures and dislocations of the elbow. In: Rockwood CA Jr, Green DP, Bucholz RW, et al, editors. Fractures in adults. 5th edition. Philadelphia: Lippincott, Williams & Wilkins; 2001. p. 921–34.

[2] O'Driscoll SW. Elbow dislocations. In: Morey B, editor. The elbow and its disorders. 3rd edition. Philadelphia: WB Saunders; 2000. p. 409–20.

[3] O'Driscoll SW, Morrey BF. Elbow dislocation and subluxation: a spectrum of instability. Clin Orthop Relat Res 1992;280:186–97.

[4] Cohen MS, Hastings HH. Acute elbow dislocation: evaluation and management. J Am Acad Orthop Surg 1998;6:15–23.

[5] Melhoff T. The elbow dislocation revisited: pathoanatomy, stabilizing structures, and keys to rehabilitation. In: Morrey BF, editor. Current concepts of elbow surgery, a comprehensive review. Rosemont (IL): American Academy of Orthopaedic Surgeons; 1992. p. 76–83.

[6] Melhoff TL, Noble PC, Bennett JB, et al. Simple dislocation of the elbow in the adult: results after closed treatment. J Bone Joint Surg Am 1988;70:244–9.

[7] Josefsson PO, Gentz CF, Johnell O, et al. Surgical versus non-surgical treatment of ligamentous injuries following dislocation of the elbow joint. J Bone Joint Surg Am 1987;69:605–8.

[8] Matev I. A radiological sign of entrapment of the median nerve in the elbow joint after posterior dislocation: a report of two cases. J Bone Joint Surg Br 1976;58:353–7.

[9] Ross G, McDevitt ER, Chronister R, et al. Treatment of simple elbow dislocation using an immediate motion protocol. Am J Sports Med 1999;27:308–11.

Orthop Clin N Am 39 (2008) 163–171

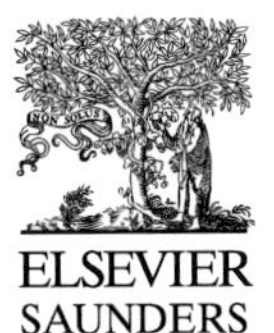

ELSEVIER
SAUNDERS

ORTHOPEDIC
CLINICS
OF NORTH AMERICA

Pediatric Supracondylar Fractures and Pediatric Physeal Elbow Fractures

M. Wade Shrader, MD

The CORE Institute, 2730 W. Agua Fria Freeway, Suite 103, Phoenix, AZ 85027, USA

Elbow fractures in children are extremely common, making up approximately 15% of all fractures in pediatric patients. Pediatric elbow fractures make up a much larger proportion of operative fractures in children, however, being as high as 85% in some series [1]. The unique radiographic anatomy of the pediatric elbow, along with the potential for neurovascular compromise, often provokes anxiety in orthopedic surgeons. A thorough understanding of the anatomy and treatment principles makes the care for these children more straightforward, however. The distal humerus makes up approximately 85% of all elbow fractures in children. The most common fractures of the distal humerus in children are supracondylar humerus fractures, lateral condyle fractures, medial epicondyle fractures, and transphyseal humerus fractures. Each of these fractures is discussed in detail, outlining their radiographic features, principles of treatment, and potential complications.

Evaluation of the pediatric patient

Care of the pediatric patient who has an elbow fracture must begin with a thorough and timely physical examination. This examination is often difficult because of pain and anxiety, especially with very small children. A gentle approach with the child and parent is always best. By starting with a complete examination of the uninjured extremity, the child can be shown that the examination will not be painful.

Examination of the injured extremity begins with inspection. Often, the displaced, type III supracondylar fracture has a characteristic deformity. The cubital fossa is checked for any

tenting of the skin that would indicate that the fracture has punctured through the brachialis, which would be a much more difficult reduction. Lateral condyle fractures, however, usually have little deformity, but have swelling located laterally with more ecchymoses than other elbow fractures. Signs and symptoms of compartment syndrome, a rare but devastating complication in children, must be ruled out.

The neurovascular examination is critical. Many children are hesitant to complete a motor examination, but every effort should be made to make a complete assessment. In particular, finger flexion should be assessed for a possible anterior interosseous nerve (AIN) palsy, and that should be documented preoperatively. Most children should be able to provide a good sensory examination in all three nerve distributions: medial, radial, and ulnar nerves.

Although the radial pulse should be checked, the overall viability and capillary refill are the most important aspects of the vascular examination. Many children who have displaced supracondylar humerus fractures do not have a palpable radial pulse. These pulses often return after closed reduction. If the child has a pink, warm hand with good capillary refill, a vascular injury is unlikely. These children can be splinted and treated urgently, often the next day. The child who has a cold, pale hand with poor capillary refill is obviously a surgical emergency and needs to be taken to the operating room immediately.

Basic radiography and ossification of the pediatric elbow

Radiographs of pediatric elbow fractures are difficult to interpret because most of the child's

---

E-mail address: wade.shrader@thecoreinstitute.com

elbow is nonossified cartilage at the typical age for distal humerus fractures. The growth centers in children appear in a predictable fashion based on the child's age and gender [2]. The knowledge of when these growth centers appear is crucial to the accurate interpretation of pediatric elbow fracture radiographs and appropriate treatment decisions. In general, the ossification rate for girls is greater than that for boys; however, there can be individual variations.

The capitellum is the first ossification center to appear, and usually is well formed by the age of 1 year in both boys and girls. The radial head then follows at about 5 to 6 years of age. The medial epicondyle often appears during this time frame, slightly lagging behind the appearance of the radial head. The olecranon is next, which appears between 8 and 10 years of age. That is followed by the trochlea, and finally the lateral epicondyle.

As in all areas of orthopedics, radiograph assessment must be made with two, true orthogonal views. This statement is especially true because of the unossified anatomy and inherent difficulty in interpreting these radiographs. Obtaining these true lateral radiographs can be difficult in a child who has just been injured and has a large amount of pain. Nevertheless, the orthopedic surgeon must have good views to make the appropriate and accurate diagnosis. Occasionally, oblique radiographs can be helpful, especially in diagnosing subtle lateral condyle fractures and assessing displacement.

The anterior humeral line and the capitellum are the cornerstones to proper interpretation of pediatric elbow fractures. The anterior humeral line should bisect the capitellum on the lateral radiograph. The radial head should point toward the capitellum on all views; if this is not true, then there may be a lateral condyle fracture or a dislocation of the radial head (as in a Monteggia fracture).

The Baumann angle is another important parameter in children's elbow radiographs. It is the angle between the physeal line of the lateral condyle of the humerus and a line perpendicular to the long axis of the humeral shaft. The normal angle is between 8 and 28 degrees, with the large spread indicating large subject-to-subject variations. A very small Baumann angle is a warning to the orthopedic surgeon that a varus deformity exists.

The fat-pad signs are always discussed and often confused when considering pediatric elbow fractures [3,4]. Fat pads are most useful in diagnosing occult, nondisplaced, or minimally displaced fractures. Most children who do not have an injury have an anterior fat-pad sign; this is simply the anterior elbow capsule displacing the brachialis. If this fat pad is enlarged, the so-called "sail sign," the child usually has an osseous injury. A posterior fat-pad sign is almost always found in children who have fractures; the literature shows a 75% sensitivity for fracture.

Supracondylar humerus fractures

Supracondylar humerus fractures are the most common elbow fracture in children (between 50% and 70%) [5]. They typically occur in children 3 to 10 years of age and are more common in males. The mechanism of injury is usually an extension force on the distal humerus causing an extension-type fracture (95%); this usually happens with a fall onto an outstretched hand. These falls can occur while running, playing sports, or much more commonly on playground equipment or from trampolines. More rarely a flexion-type supracondylar humerus fracture may occur with a direct blow to the elbow with the elbow flexed. The relatively high potential for neurovascular compromise and residual deformity make the pediatric supracondylar humerus fracture a serious injury [6].

Displaced supracondylar humerus fractures usually have an obvious deformity and swelling on physical examination. Minimally displaced fractures can be difficult to detect on either physical examination or radiographs, however. A thorough physical examination is critical, concentrating on the neurovascular examination. These fractures have a 10% to 15% neurologic injury rate, usually an AIN palsy [7]. A compartment syndrome should be ruled out. Extreme pain (more pain than typical for a child who has a fracture), pain with passive range of motion of the distal fingers (distal interphalangeal and proximal interphalangeal joints), and a full, tense compartment are the most reliable signs. The vascular examination is equally important, with many of these children having diminished radial pulses. The literature has shown that children who have brisk capillary refill and pink, warm hands are not likely to have any permanent vascular injury. A child who has a cold and cyanotic hand represents a surgical emergency.

The differential diagnosis includes a lateral condyle fracture, a transphyseal distal humerus fracture (especially in younger children), and an elbow dislocation. A true elbow dislocation is rare in children, however, and a report of that should be viewed with some suspicion.

Most displaced supracondylar humerus fractures are extension-type injuries. The less common flexion-type fracture only occurs in 2% of the fractures. The Gartland classification system is used for extension-type supracondylar humerus fractures. A type I fracture is essentially a nondisplaced fracture. These injuries can be difficult to detect on radiographs. A positive posterior fat-pad sign is often present even when a radiolucent fracture line is not seen.

A type II fracture still has the posterior periosteum intact connecting the distal fragment and the humeral shaft. The anterior humeral line is anterior to the capitellum and does not intersect. The fracture often appears to be hinged posteriorly. In contrast, the type III supracondylar humerus fracture has a complete displacement of the distal fragment relative to the humeral shaft with fractures of both cortices, and there is often significant displacement. With proper radiographs, the diagnosis of this fracture is not difficult to make.

A complete radiographic assessment of a child who has a supracondylar humerus fracture must include radiographs of the forearm. There is a 10% to 15% chance of an ipsilateral concurrent distal radius for forearm fracture in these children.

Treatment of type I fractures is fairly straightforward. These children should be splinted on the day of injury with a long-arm posterior splint and side gutters, usually neutral rotation and in 90 degrees of elbow flexion. The child returns in approximately 1 week, and the splint is exchanged for a long-arm cast if the fracture has remained nondisplaced. After an additional 2 to 3 weeks of immobilization, the cast is removed and the child begins range-of-motion exercises.

Displaced fractures always require a reduction to decrease the risk for cosmetic deformities and poor functional outcomes. Although some reports favor reduction and casting (in hyperflexion) of type II supracondylar fractures, we believe that there is additional risk with this technique, both in neurovascular compromise and in losing adequate reduction. The preferred treatment of all type II and type III fractures at our institution is closed reduction and percutaneous pinning in the operating room under complete sterile conditions (Fig. 1 A, B) [8–11].

The reduction is performed with longitudinal traction followed by correction of the coronal plane (varus/valgus) deformity. The elbow is then

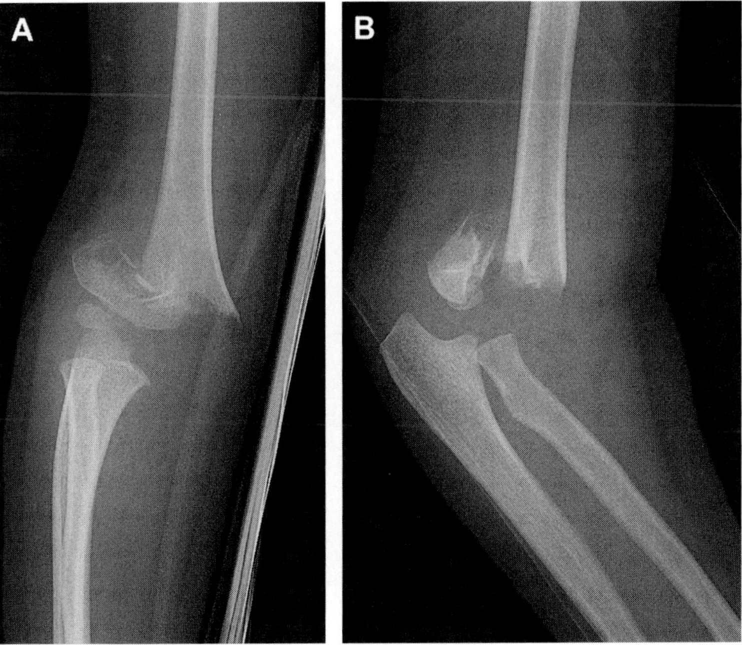

Fig. 1. (*A, B*) A 3-year-old boy status post fall out of bed onto his right upper extremity.

hyperflexed accompanied by direct anterior pressure over the olecranon to complete the reduction. Keeping the elbow in a hyperflexed position, lateral and oblique radiographs are used to assess the reduction. Once satisfactory, a lateral pin is placed in a retrograde fashion from distal lateral to proximal medial, with care taken to ensure bicortical purchase. Once the initial pin is in, the elbow is brought into more extension for an anteroposterior (AP) and lateral radiograph. If the reduction and pin position are satisfactory, then an additional lateral pin is placed in a divergent fashion. The elbow is then ranged slightly under live fluoroscopy, with a lateral view. If there is any instability of the construct with this maneuver, a medial pin is placed for additional fracture stability (Fig. 2 A–D).

There is much debate in the literature regarding two lateral pins versus crossed pins (one lateral and one medial) [12]. Obviously, the risk with a medial pin is the ulnar nerve [13]. Biomechanical studies have shown that two crossed pins are the strongest construct. In the physiologic load range, there may not be much difference

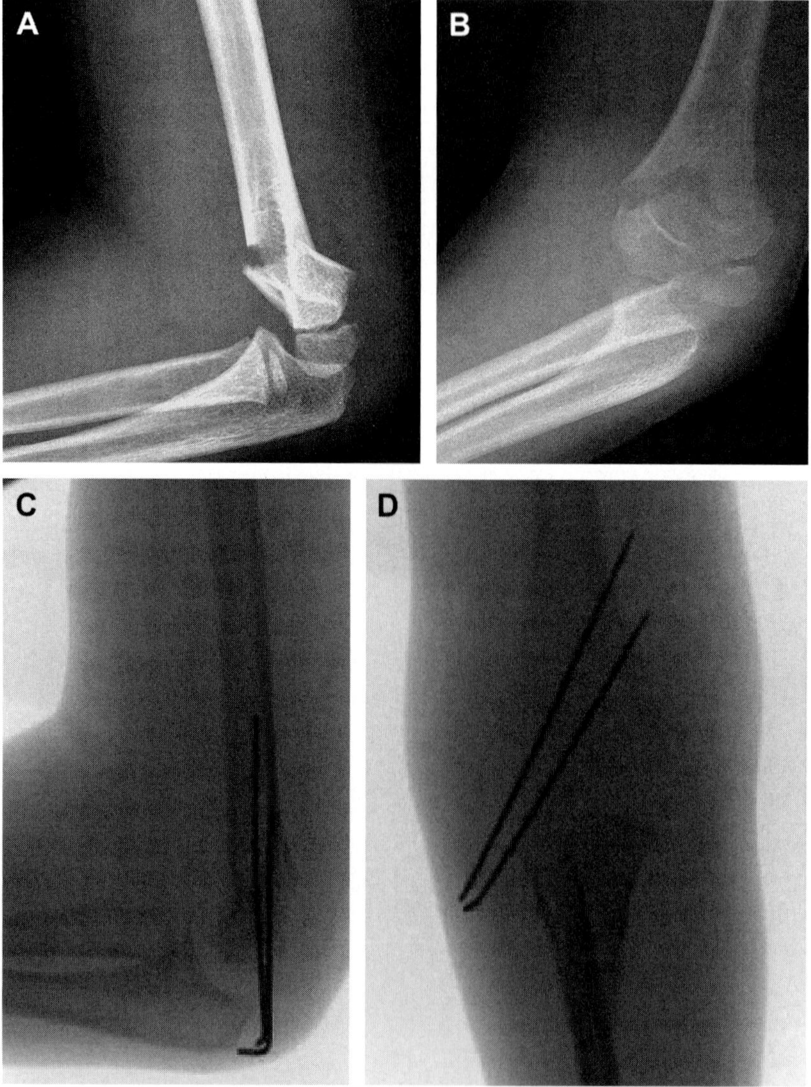

Fig. 2. (*A*, *B*) A 7-year-old boy status post fall from a fence onto his left upper extremity. (*C*, *D*) Status post closed reduction and percutaneous pinning.

between the two methods. We have found that two lateral pins, placed divergently in both planes, with good bony purchase in both fragments, is usually adequate for fracture stability. If there is any question of the stability of the construct, we simply add the medial pin. The technique for medial pin placement varies from percutaneous placement to mini-open techniques. We extend the elbow slightly to allow the ulnar nerve to displace posteriorly from the medial epicondyle. A free pin is then placed down to the anterior aspect of the medial epicondyle. The driver is then placed over the pin, and it is driven across the fracture site. If there is a new postoperative ulnar nerve palsy, the pin is removed in the recovery room.

The pins are bent and cut; sterile dressings are applied and the patient is placed in a long-arm splint with a lateral gutter in about 80 degrees of flexion. Patients who have type III fractures are kept overnight for neurovascular observation. Patients return in 1 week for radiographs in the office to rule out fracture displacement. If the splint remains fairly pristine, we overwrap the splint and keep the child in this for an additional 2 to 3 weeks. If the splint is worn, we change the child over to a long-arm cast. When the child returns at the next visit, the pins are removed in the office, and range-of-motion exercises are begun.

Early complications of supracondylar fractures usually are attributable to neurovascular compromise. The literature reports a wide variation in the incidence of vascular compromise in these patients [14]. Obviously, a child who has a cold and cyanotic hand represents a surgical emergency. These children should have an emergent reduction done in the emergency room. Hyperflexion of the elbow should not be done in the emergency room because this may further occlude the brachial artery. The elbow should be allowed to rest in extension, and direct anterior forward pressure is placed on the distal fragment. If this does not improve the vascular status, a vascular surgeon competent in pediatric cases should be immediately consulted for a possible exploration and revascularization.

Many times perfusion returns after adequate reduction and pinning in the operating room. The radial pulse may be absent still, however, even in the case of a pink, warm hand with good capillary refill. As in other areas, there are wide differences in opinion about how to manage these patients. We believe that a hand that is well perfused, even without a radial pulse, warrants close observation, and we usually do not obtain a vascular consultation at that point. Almost all of these children do

well without a significant vascular complication. If the child's hand is still cold and cyanotic even after reduction and pinning, vascular surgery must be consulted emergently.

Although the rate of peripheral nerve injury is as much as 15%, most of these injuries resolve in time, spontaneously improving [15,16]. An accurate, thorough preoperative and postoperative assessment and documentation of the neurologic status of these children is crucial [17]. Compartment syndrome, or Volkmann ischemic contracture, is always a concern in these patients. Frequent neurovascular monitoring and emergent fasciotomies often preclude the devastating consequences of this complication [18,19].

The most common complication of supracondylar fractures is malunion, usually cubitus varus [20]. This deformity arises because of rotational malposition, usually in posteromedially displaced fractures. Every attempt should be made to avoid this complication at the time of reduction. Problems arising from this malunion are primarily cosmetic, because a varus carrying angle at the elbow is very noticeable. Functional deficits are uncommon. Unlike other malunions in children, there is little remodeling potential in the distal humerus. Treatment of this complication is therefore a supracondylar osteotomy [21].

Stiffness after supracondylar humerus fractures is extremely rare. We typically assess range of motion 6 to 8 weeks after immobilization is discontinued. It is the rare child who does not have full range of motion with normal function at this follow-up visit.

Lateral condyle fractures

Lateral condyle fractures are the second most common operative elbow fracture in children [22]. Lateral condyle fractures usually occur as a result of a fall on an outstretched hand, with a similar age distribution to supracondylar humerus fractures. These fractures are notoriously difficult to diagnose. Fractures with minimal displacement are difficult to see radiographically. Displaced fractures are often misdiagnosed as supracondylar humerus fractures by emergency room physicians. Most of these fractures are displaced, intra-articular fractures; as such, they often require open reduction to anatomically reduce the articular surface.

As in all cases, the physical examination should have a thorough neurovascular examination. The risk for neurovascular compromise in a lateral condyle fracture is much lower than that of a supracondylar humerus fracture, however. Many patients who have a lateral condyle fracture have more ecchymoses laterally, because the tearing of the lateral intermuscular septum causes subcutaneous bleeding.

True AP and lateral radiographs make the diagnosis much easier. For minimally displaced fractures, however, even a complete two-view elbow series may not be adequate. For these cases, oblique radiographs may be necessary. For displaced fractures, the diagnosis is confirmed radiographically by the lack of a normal capitellum–radial head relationship; in these fractures, the lateral condyle and capitellum are displaced laterally in relation to the radial head.

The Milch classification system is used for discussing lateral condyle fractures. A type I fracture extends through the ossification center of the capitellum, entering the joint lateral to the trochlear groove. Some have described this as a Salter-Harris IV fracture. A type II fracture extends medial to the trochlear groove, making the humeral-ulnar joint less stable. The most important determination is whether the fracture is displaced or nondisplaced.

Only the truly nondisplaced fractures should be treated nonoperatively [23]. These patients should be splinted with a posterior splint and lateral gutter. The patients are seen 1 week later; if the fracture remains nondisplaced, the splint is exchanged for a long-arm cast. It is imperative that these patients are seen weekly and followed with serial radiographs. One pitfall in taking care of children who have lateral condyle fractures is the missed late displacement that often occurs in these minimally displaced fractures. We use oblique radiographs at each follow-up in addition to the two-view elbow series. After 4 weeks of immobilization, range-of-motion exercises are begun.

Any displaced fracture is treated with open reduction and percutaneous pinning [24–26]. Recent literature has suggested the use of percutaneous pinning and arthrograms to verify reduction of the articular surface [27]. It has been this author's experience that the true displacement seen on open exploration is much greater than that appreciated on a radiograph. In our institution, therefore, all displaced lateral condyle fractures are treated with open reduction [28].

A lateral approach is made to the elbow. The fracture has usually done most of the dissection; blunt dissection through the torn lateral fascia

usually leads right down to the fracture. It is important to dissect medially through the joint and divide any synovial attachments to the displaced fragment. Furthermore, the fragment should be displaced and thoroughly irrigated to remove hematoma and fibrinous debris. Any dissection needing to be done on the lateral epicondyle and metaphysis should be anterior, to avoid the posterior blood supply and minimize the risk for avascular necrosis. The displaced fragment is reduced under direct visualization, often with the aid of a reduction clamp, "joystick" Kirschner (K)–wires, or the assistant's manual pressure. Percutaneous pins (0.062 K-wires) are then placed in a divergent fashion.

Postoperatively, the patient is splinted and followed as a supracondylar humerus fracture. We typically leave these pins in until evidence of radiographic healing is present, which is typically 4 to 6 weeks. The pins are then removed and range-of-motion exercises are begun (Fig. 3 A–D).

The most common complications following lateral condyle fractures include nonunion, cubitus varus/valgus, and fishtail deformity [29]. Nonunions are especially rare in pediatric patients; however, the lateral condyle of the distal humerus is one area that is particularly prone to nonunion. Many theories have been suggested for the cause of this, including posterior dissection and disruption of blood flow or the presence of synovial fluid inhibiting fracture healing. One of the most important aspects of treating these fractures is meticulous surgical technique that avoids the risk for nonunion. Furthermore, these patients should be followed closely until radiographic healing has occurred.

Nonunion often presents with cubitus valgus, as the fracture fragment drifts into valgus without healing to the metaphysis. This complication often presents with a tardy ulnar nerve palsy from a stretch phenomenon on the nerve from the increase in carrying angle. Treatment of this is focused on treatment of the nonunion. For the true nonunion, often healing can be achieved with an open reduction and screw fixation.

Cubitus varus is the most common complication in lateral condyle fractures, occurring as a malunion, growth arrest, or combination. Varus following lateral condyle fractures is rarely as big a problem as when it occurs in supracondylar humerus fractures. Most times, a little parental reassurance is all that is needed. The dreaded fishtail deformity is also a rare complication that arises from avascular necrosis of the distal

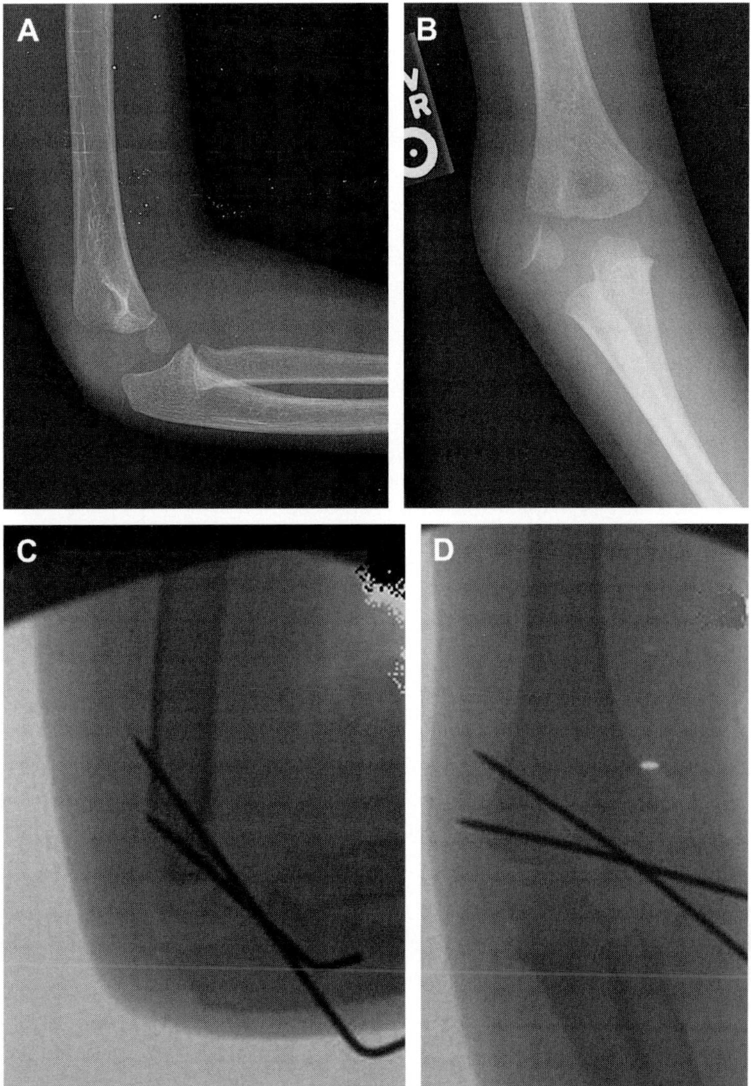

Fig. 3. (*A*, *B*) A 4-year-old girl status post fall from monkey bars onto her right upper extremity. (*C*, *D*) Status post closed reduction and percutaneous pinning.

fragment; however, growth arrests may also contribute.

Medial epicondyle fracture

Medial epicondyle fractures are also relatively common injuries in pediatric patients, accounting for 10% of all children's elbow fractures. The typical age is between 7 and 15 years, and 50% of these fractures are associated with elbow dislocations [30]. The injury occurs from a valgus stress producing an avulsion-type fracture from pull of the flexor-pronator muscle groups. The injury may occur from falls producing the deforming force or from sports activity (ie, throwing a baseball) [31].

The child typically presents with a flexed elbow and tenderness directly over the medial aspect of the arm. Ulnar nerve paresthesias may be present. In throwing athletes, there is often a history of a popping sound, with severe pain immediately following.

Minimally displaced fractures may be difficult to appreciate with radiographs. Often, comparison films with the contralateral, normal extremity demonstrate the increased displacement of the injured medial epicondyle. Markedly displaced fractures are usually easier to identify. In the case of an elbow dislocation, an incarcerated fragment in the ulnar-humeral joint may be present. If the radiographs do not show a medial epicondyle in a child older than 7 years of age, a close inspection of the film should be made to see if the fragment is in the elbow joint. Many times, with a younger patient, the medial epicondyle is not completely ossified; a noncentrically reduced ulnohumeral joint on the lateral radiograph may be the only clue that the fragment is in the elbow joint.

Most pediatric orthopedic surgeons treat minimally displaced (<5 mm) medial epicondyle fractures with conservative care [32]. The patient is originally placed in a long-arm splint for 1 to 2 weeks, followed by range-of-motion exercises. The patient and parents are reassured that most children do extremely well with this fracture, but they are warned that radiographic union may not occur (fibrous union).

Treatment of the displaced fragment that is incarcerated in the ulnohumeral joint always requires reduction [33]. A single attempt is made to reduce the fragment with closed means, by opening the joint with a valgus stress, supinating the forearm, and stretching the finger and wrist flexors. If this maneuver is not successful, we proceed to open reduction and screw fixation of the fragment. Ulnar nerve transposition should always accompany an open reduction of the displaced medial epicondyle.

Treatment of nonincarcerated displaced fractures is more controversial. The literature has several series of excellent results with nonoperative management. These fractures may only result in a fibrous union, but the patients rarely have functional deficits. There have also been recent reports in the literature of excellent results following open reduction and internal fixation [34]. We reserve surgery for those patients who are competitive athletes and those for whom minor elbow instability may cause significant issues in the future.

Complications from medial epicondyle fractures are rare, but include stiffness, ulnar neuritis, and symptomatic nonunion. It is important to begin early range-of-motion exercises in these patients to prevent elbow stiffness. The incidence of ulnar nerve symptoms varies from 10% to 15%. Symptomatic nonunion should be initially treated with an attempt at osteosynthesis with internal fixation. Recalcitrant nonunions may be treated with fragment excision and medial collateral ligament reconstruction.

Transphyseal elbow fractures

Transphyseal fractures of the distal humerus are relatively rare, but they present a unique diagnostic challenge [35,36]. These injuries typically occur in children 2 years of age or less, before the appearance of the capitellum ossification center. In children so young, the entire distal humerus is made up of cartilage, so a direct visualization of the fracture on radiographs is often not seen. In fact, these injuries are often described as elbow dislocations, an extremely rare injury in a child less than 3 years old. Furthermore, this injury is a result of nonaccidental trauma (child abuse) in more than half of the cases. The mechanism of injury is either a fall on an outstretched extremity or a rotatory mechanism in those cases of abuse. Neurovascular compromise is rare in these patients.

This injury requires a careful and knowledgeable assessment of the radiographs. The key to this assessment is the radial head–capitellum relationship. In a true elbow dislocation, the radial head no longer points toward the capitellum. A transphyseal elbow fracture initially appears like a dislocation; the radius and ulna do not align with the humerus. In the transphyseal fracture, however, the capitellum is still aligned with the radial head, especially evident on the AP view. This fracture may be difficult to assess in the extremely young child, when the capitellar ossification center has not yet appeared. In these cases, either an MRI or an arthrogram may be necessary for the diagnosis.

The treatment of displaced transphyseal fractures is similar to supracondylar humerus fractures: closed reduction and percutaneous pinning. Arthrography is used intraoperatively for these patients, because of the difficulty visualizing the distal humeral anatomy in children so young. The postoperative management is identical to that of the supracondylar humerus fracture.

References

[1] Wilkins KE, Rockwood CA Jr. Fractures and dislocations of the elbow region. In: Wilkins KE, Beaty JH, editors. Fractures in children. 4th edition. Philadelphia: Lippincott-Raven; 1996. p. 653–904.

[2] Cheng JC, Wing-Man K, Shen WY, et al. A new look at the sequential development of elbow-ossification centers in children. J Pediatr Orthop 1998; 18:161–7.

[3] Corbett RH. Displaced fat pads in trauma to the elbow. Injury 1978;9:297–8.

[4] Skaggs DL, Mirzayan R. The posterior fat pad sign in association with occult fracture of the elbow in children. J Bone Joint Surg Am 1999;81:1429–33.

[5] Alburger PD, Weidner PL, Randal RB. Supracondylar fractures of the humerus in children. J Pediatr Orthop 1992;12:16–9.

[6] Boyd DW, Aronson DD. Supracondylar fractures of the humerus: a prospective study of percutaneous pinning. J Pediatr Orthop 1992;12:789–94.

[7] Campbell CC, Waters PM, Emans JB, et al. Neurovascular injury and displacement in type III supracondylar humerus fractures. J Pediatr Orthop 1995;15:47–52.

[8] Cheng J, Lam T, Shen W. Closed reduction and percutaneous pinning for type III displaced supracondylar fractures of the humerus in children. J Orthop Trauma 1995;9:511–5.

[9] Pirone AM, Graham HK, Krajbich JI. Management of displaced extension-type supracondylar fractures of the humerus in children. J Bone Joint Surg Am 1988;70:641–50.

[10] Weiland AJ, Meyer S, Tolo VT, et al. Surgical treatment of displaced supracondylar fractures of the humerus in children. J Bone Joint Surg Am 1978; 60:657–61.

[11] Iyengar S, Hoffinger S, Townsend D. Early versus delayed reduction and pinning of type III displaced supracondylar fractures of the humerus in children: a comparative study. J Orthop Trauma 1999;13: 51–5.

[12] Zionts LE, McKellop HA, Hathaway R. Torsional strength of pin configurations used to fix supracondylar fractures of the humerus in children. J Bone Joint Surg Am 1994;76:253–6.

[13] Lyons J, Ashley E, Hoffer M. Ulnar nerve palsies after percutaneous cross-pinning of supracondylar fractures in children's elbows. J Pediatr Orthop 1998;18:43–5.

[14] Schoenecker P, Delgado E, Rotman M, et al. Pulseless arm in association with totally displaced supracondylar fracture. J Orthop Trauma 1996;10:410–5.

[15] Bailey GG Jr. Nerve injuries in supracondylar fractures of the humerus in children. N Engl J Med 1939;221:260–3.

[16] Cramer KE, Green NE, DeVito DP. Incidence of anterior interosseous nerve palsy in supracondylar humerus fractures in children. J Pediatr Orthop 1993;13:502–5.

[17] McGraw JJ, Akbarnia BA, Hanel DP, et al. Neurological complications resulting from supracondylar fractures of the humerus in children. J Pediatr Orthop 1986;6:647–50.

[18] Mubarak SJ, Carroll NC. Volkmann's contracture in children: aetiology and prevention. J Bone Joint Surg Br 1979;61:285–93.

[19] Blount WP. Volkmann's ischemic contracture. Surg Gynecol Obstet 1950;90:244–6.

[20] Gaddy BC, Manske PR, Pruitt DL, et al. Distal humeral osteotomy for correction of posttraumatic cubitus varus. J Pediatr Orthop 1994;14:214–9.

[21] Graham B, Tredwell SJ, Beauchamp RD, et al. Supracondylar osteotomy of the humerus for correction of cubitus varus. J Pediatr Orthop 1990;10:228–31.

[22] Beaty JH. Fractures and dislocations about the elbow in children. Instr Course Lect 1992;41:373–84.

[23] Bast SC, Hoffer MM, Aval S. Nonoperative treatment for minimally and nondisplaced lateral humeral condyle fractures in children. J Pediatr Orthop 1998;18:448–50.

[24] Rutherford AJ. Fractures of the lateral humeral condyle in children. J Bone Joint Surg Am 1985;67:851–6.

[25] Foster DE, Sullivan JA, Gross RH. Lateral humeral condylar fractures in children. J Pediatr Orthop 1985;5:16–22.

[26] Badelon O, Bensahel H, Mazda K, et al. Lateral humeral condylar fractures in children: a report of 47 cases. J Pediatr Orthop 1988;8:31–4.

[27] Mintzer CM, Water PM, Brown DJ, et al. Percutaneous pinning in the treatment of displaced lateral condyle fractures. J Pediatr Orthop 1994;14:462–5.

[28] Herring JA. Lateral condylar fracture of the elbow. J Pediatr Orthop 1986;6:724–7.

[29] Flynn JC, Richards JF. Non-union of minimally displaced fractures of the lateral condyle of humerus in children. J Bone Joint Surg Am 1971;53:1096–101.

[30] Fowles JV, Slimane N, Kassab MT. Elbow dislocation with avulsion of the medial humeral epicondyle. J Bone Joint Surg Br 1990;72:102–4.

[31] Diass JJ, Johnson GV, Hoskinson J, et al. Management of severely displaced medial epicondyle fractures. J Orthop Trauma 1987;1:59–62.

[32] Josefsson PO, Danielsson LG. Epicondylar elbow fracture in children: 35-year follow-up of 56 unreduced cases. Acta Orthop Scand 1986;57:313–31.

[33] Wilson JN. Treatment of fractures of the medial epicondyle of the humerus. J Bone Joint Surg 1960;43: 778–81.

[34] Hines RF, Herndon WA, Evans JP. Operative treatment of medial epicondyle fractures in children. Clin Orthop 1987;221:170–4.

[35] DeLee JC, Wilkins KE, Rogers LF, et al. Fracture separation of the distal humeral epiphysis. J Bone Joint Surg Am 1980;67:46–51.

[36] Barrett WP, Almquist EA, Staheli LT. Fracture separation of the distal humeral physis in the newborn. J Pediatr Orthop 1984;4:617–9.

Orthop Clin N Am 39 (2008) 173–185

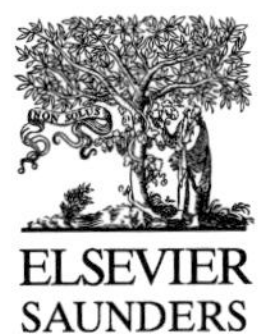

ORTHOPEDIC
CLINICS
OF NORTH AMERICA

Current Recommendations for the Treatment of Radial Head Fractures

Yishai Rosenblatt, MD, George S. Athwal, MD, FRCSC,
Kenneth J. Faber, MD, MHPE, FRCSC*

*Hand and Upper Limb Centre, St. Joseph's Health Care, University of Western Ontario,
268 Grosvenor Street, London, Ontario, Canada N6A 4L6*

Radial head fractures are the most common type of elbow fractures. These fractures can occur in isolation or be associated with other elbow fractures and ligament injuries. Associated injuries include coronoid fractures, distal humerus articular shear fractures, Monteggia's fractures, and disruption of the collateral ligaments, interosseous ligaments, or both [1–3].

Although a consensus has emerged that favors the nonsurgical treatment of undisplaced fractures [4], controversy surrounds the treatment of displaced radial head fractures [5]. Options for the treatment of displaced fractures include nonoperative management, fragment excision [6,7], whole head excision [8–10], open reduction and internal fixation (ORIF) [11–15], and radial head arthroplasty [16–22].

The purpose of this article is to review the mechanisms that result in radial head fracture, to describe important physical findings that assist in identifying injuries associated with radial head fractures, and to define the role of the various interventions described for the treatment of radial head fractures.

Mechanism of injury, symptoms, and signs

Elbow stability is maintained by the complex interplay among articular surfaces, ligaments, and muscles. The radial head is an important valgus stabilizer of the elbow, particularly in the setting of an incompetent medial collateral ligament,

which is the primary stabilizer against valgus force [23–26]. The radial head is also an important axial stabilizer of the forearm and resists varus and posterolateral rotatory instability by tensioning the lateral collateral ligament [27,28]. In addition, up to 60% of the load transfer across the elbow occurs through the radiocapitellar articulation [29].

Radial head fractures typically result from a fall on the outstretched arm. Axial, valgus, and posterolateral rotational patterns of loading are all thought to be potentially responsible for these fractures (Fig. 1A–C). An axial force applied to the wrist is transmitted proximally and can exit through the radial head. In addition to radial head fractures, rupture of the interosseous ligament of the forearm can lead to complex injury patterns such as the Essex-Lopresti injury [30,31]. When a valgus force is applied to the elbow, the radial head can fail in compression, with resultant medial collateral ligament rupture. The final injury mechanism is associated with posterolateral rotatory instability. As the lateral collateral ligament complex fails, an episode of elbow subluxation can result in shear injuries of the radial head, coronoid, and distal humerus [3].

In addition to recognizing signs directly associated with an acute radial head fracture, the physical examiner should also identify signs associated with elbow or forearm instability. Inspection may reveal ecchymosis and swelling along the forearm and medial and lateral aspects of the elbow, which may correspond to associated ligamentous injuries. Careful palpation of the radial head, distal humerus, proximal ulna, medial and lateral collateral ligaments of the elbow, the

---

* Corresponding author.
E-mail address: kjfaber@uwo.ca (K.J. Faber).

0030-5898/08/$ - see front matter © 2008 Elsevier Inc. All rights reserved.
doi:10.1016/j.ocl.2007.12.008

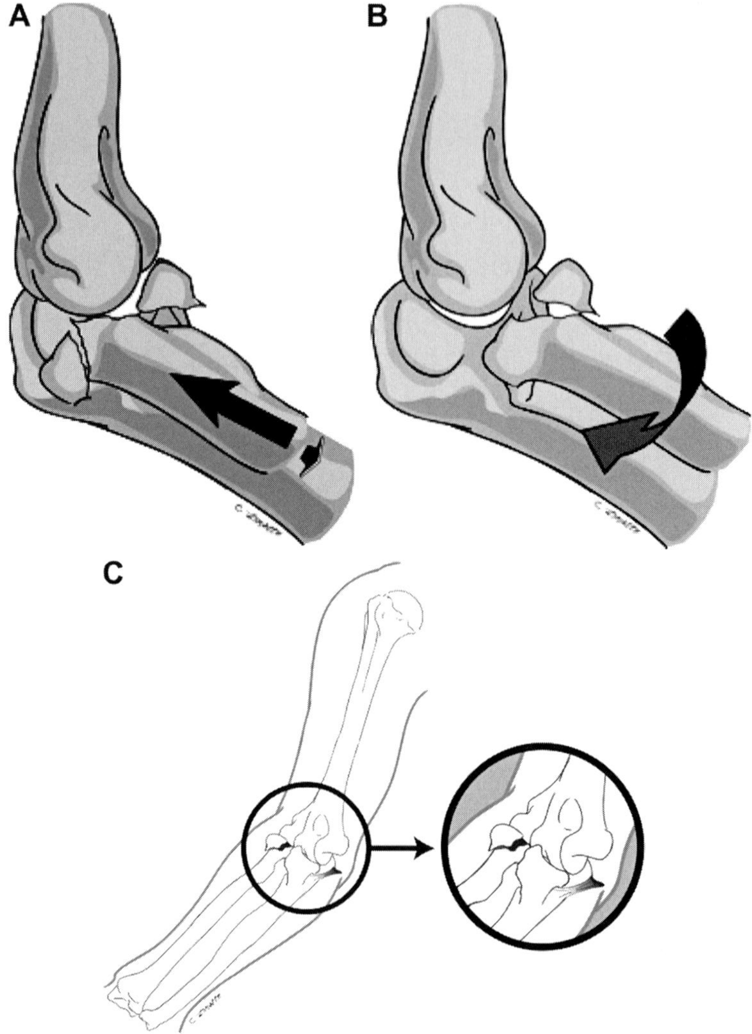

Fig. 1. (*A*) A fall on an outstretched hand transmits an axial load to the elbow. The energy can be dissipated through a fracture of the radial head. (*B*) Failure of the lateral collateral ligament complex results in posterolateral rotatory instability of the elbow. During the episode of instability the radial head can be fractured. (*C*) Failure of the medial collateral ligament results in valgus instability of the elbow and subsequent compression of the radial head.

interosseous ligament of the forearm, and the distal radioulnar joint should be performed in addition to careful examination of the adjacent joints such as the shoulder and wrist. Elbow range of motion (ROM) including forearm rotation should be evaluated, and the presence of crepitus or a block to motion should be noted. Aspiration of the hemarthrosis and intra-articular injection of local anesthetic is helpful in determining whether restricted motion is a consequence of pain or a true mechanical block to motion. A careful vascular and neurologic assessment of

radial, median, and ulnar nerves should be performed.

Imaging

Anteroposterior, lateral, and oblique elbow radiographs, with the x-ray beam centered on the radiocapitellar joint, usually provide sufficient information for the diagnosis and treatment of radial head fractures. If the biceps tuberosity is included in the radiographs, then the relationship of the fracture to the radius shaft can often be determined. This information is helpful when planning surgical exposures.

Bilateral posteroanterior radiographs of both wrists in neutral rotation should be performed when the clinical examination reveals forearm or ulnar-sided wrist pain that is suggestive of injury to the interosseous ligament. The ulnar variance should be evaluated because there is a higher incidence of an associated interosseous ligament injury in this group of patients [1].

CT with sagittal, coronal, and three-dimensional reconstructions may assist with preoperative planning and can help the surgeon predict whether a displaced radial head fracture can be treated with ORIF or whether an arthroplasty is needed.

Classification

Mason [32] classified radial head fractures as type I, fissure or marginal sector fractures without displacement; type II, marginal sector fractures with displacement; or type III, comminuted fractures involving the whole head. Mason's original classification was subsequently modified by Johnston [33] with the addition of a fourth type, a radial head fracture associated with an elbow dislocation. Morrey [34] further modified Mason's classification by including radial neck fractures and stratifying fractures based on significant articular segment displacement (>2 mm) and fragment size ($\geq$30% of the articular surface).

Hotchkiss [35] applied management guidelines to the Mason classification for radial head fractures. Type I fractures are minimally displaced and can be treated nonsurgically. Type II fractures are displaced greater than 2 mm or block normal forearm rotation and can be successfully treated with ORIF. Type III fractures are comminuted, not amenable to ORIF, and treated with excision or arthroplasty. Although these guidelines help with intraoperative decision making, they do not provide preoperative criteria to determine the fracture type or guidelines for treatment. Mason's classification remains the most widely used in clinical practice, even though it has been shown to have poor to moderate intra- and inter-observer reliability [36].

Treatment options

Important factors to consider when making treatment decisions include radial head fracture configuration, associated fractures, elbow and forearm ROM, and clinical or radiographic findings that suggest elbow or forearm instability. Bone quality, fragment size, comminution, impaction, and displacement influence decision making regarding the optimal management of each radial head fracture. Fragments that are displaced and interfere with elbow or forearm ROM need to be identified and treated. Clinical or radiographic findings that suggest collateral ligament instability or forearm axial instability need to be considered when developing a management plan.

Nonoperative treatment

Undisplaced or small (<33% of radial head) minimally displaced fractures (<2 mm) usually originate from the anterolateral aspect of the radial head and can be treated with early motion provided that there is no mechanical block to motion [4,37]. Aspiration of the hemarthrosis and intra-articular injection of a local anesthetic help the treating physician rule out a mechanical block, provide pain relief, and permit early ROM [38]. Treatment consists of a collar and cuff sling and initiation of active ROM exercises within 2 to 3 days as the injury discomfort subsides. ROM should improve within the first 6 weeks following the injury and often returns to a functional range within 6 to 12 weeks. In cases in which extension does not improve progressively within the first 6 weeks, nighttime static progressive extension splints may be used.

Most series report 85% to 95% good results for undisplaced fractures managed with early motion [6,39,40]. Fractures initially treated nonsurgically and remaining symptomatic can be treated with delayed excision of the fractured radial head with satisfactory results, providing that the interosseous membrane and medial collateral ligament are intact [41]. Akesson and colleagues [42] reported favorable results with conservative treatment of moderately displaced radial head fractures (Mason type II) at a mean follow-up of 19 years. The absolute amount of displacement that can be successfully treated nonsurgically with early ROM remains undefined.

Operative treatment

Surgical approaches

The patient can be positioned supine with the affected arm on an arm table, supine with a sandbag placed beneath the ipsilateral scapula to assist in positioning the arm across the chest, or in a lateral position with the affected arm held over a bolster.

A midline posterior elbow incision is made just lateral to the tip of the olecranon, and a full-thickness lateral fasciocutaneous flap is elevated on the deep fascia. This extensile incision decreases the risk of cutaneous nerve injury and provides access to the radial head, coronoid, and medial and lateral collateral ligaments for the management of more complex injuries [43,44]. Alternatively, a lateral skin incision centered over the lateral epicondyle and passing obliquely over the radial head can be used. In many circumstances, the radial head is easily visualized after opening the subcutaneous tissue due to avulsion of the lateral collateral ligament and common extensor muscles from the lateral epicondyle during the injury [45].

Splitting the extensor digitorum communis (EDC) tendon is useful for exposure of the anterior and lateral portions of the radial head. The EDC is split longitudinally at the midportion of the radial head, and the underlying radial collateral and annular ligaments are incised [35]. Dissection should remain anterior to the lateral ulnar collateral ligament to prevent iatrogenic posterolateral rotatory instability. The forearm is pronated to move the posterior interosseous nerve distally, medially, and away from the surgical approach [46,47]. The humeral origin of the radial collateral ligament and the overlying extensor muscles are elevated anteriorly off the lateral epicondyle to improve the exposure if needed.

The Kocher [48] approach is useful for exposure of the lateral and posterior portions of the radial head. The fascial interval between the extensor carpi ulnaris and anconeus muscles is identified by the diverging direction of the muscle groups and the small vascular perforators that exit at this interval. The extensor carpi ulnaris is elevated anteriorly off the lateral collateral ligament complex such that the radial collateral and annular ligaments can be incised at the midaxis of the radial head without jeopardizing elbow stability and without violating the integrity of the lateral ulnar collateral ligament. This approach provides greater protection to the posterior interosseous nerve compared to the EDC split but puts the lateral collateral ligament complex at a greater risk. Therefore, the anconeus muscle should not be elevated posteriorly.

When further exposure is required, release of the lateral collateral ligament can be considered, but careful ligament repair is required at the end of the procedure to restore varus and posterolateral rotatory stability to the elbow [27,49].

Open reduction and internal fixation

Displaced fractures that cause painful crepitus, cause restricted motion, or are associated with elbow instability patterns are managed with ORIF. Satisfactory outcomes are reported in case series when anatomic reduction and stable internal fixation is achieved [12,14,15,50]. Ikeda and colleagues [51,52] reported satisfactory and good results in patients who had comminuted Mason type III fractures of the radial head and underwent ORIF. Because the presence of greater than three fragments is associated with a greater risk of early failure of internal fixation, nonunion, and loss of forearm rotation, ORIF is not recommended in these cases [50].

As has been emphasized earlier, comminuted fractures of the radial head are often associated with a complex injury to the elbow, forearm, or both, and these additional injuries should be incorporated in to the decision making [1]. After exposing the fracture, the periosteum is usually intact over the metaphyseal fracture line, and every effort should be made to preserve the tenuous blood supply to the fragments by mobilzing them gently while using a dental pick/bone tamp/septal to the reduced anatomic position. Smooth Kirshner wires are useful as "joysticks" to reduce the fragments and for provisional fixation.

Many fixation methods and devices are described in the literature for ORIF, including standard bone screws of various sizes (2.7 mm/ 2.0 mm/1.5 mm), cannulated screws, variable pitch headless compression screws [53,54], small threaded Kirshner wires, fibrin adhesive seal [55], and absorbable pins and screws (Fig. 2A–D) [56–59]. The described fixation methods have similar reported outcomes, and no fixation method has demonstrated superiority over the other methods.

Fractures of greater complexity involving the entire head or neck require fixation that spans the head–neck junction. A number of fixation options exist, including small T- and L-shaped plates, mini condylar blade plates, locking plates, cross-cannulated screws, and precontoured anatomic radial head locking plates [60]. In noncominuted head–neck fractures, a cross-cannulated screw technique is satisfactory, whereas the presence of a neck comminution or a metaphyseal defect is best treated with plate fixation (Fig. 3A–D). If necessary, bone graft for

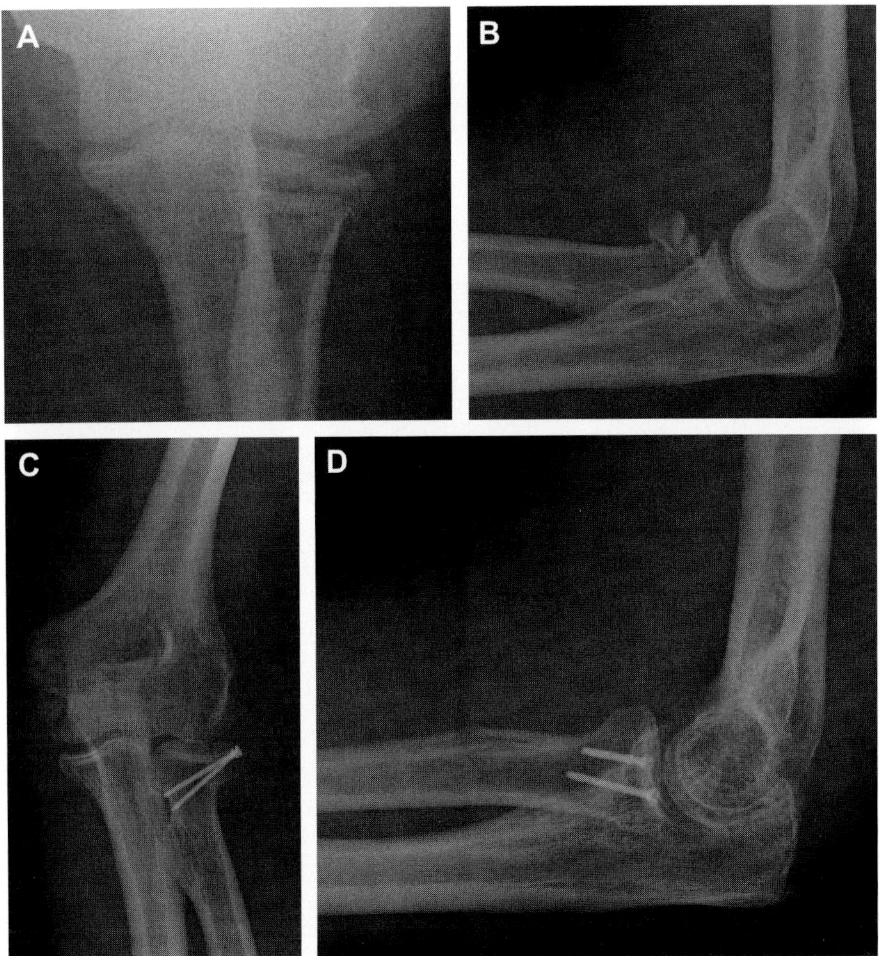

Fig. 2. Anteroposterior (*A*) and lateral (*B*) radiographs of a 48-year-old man who sustained a comminuted radial head fracture associated with an injury to the medial collateral ligament of his left elbow. (*C*, *D*) Postoperative radiographs obtained 1 year following ORIF of the radial head with two 2-mm screws and repair of the lateral collateral ligament complex. Notice the ossification at the medial aspect of the elbow.

metaphyseal defects can be obtained from the lateral epicondyle or olecranon.

Regardless of fixation technique, care should be taken to place the implants within the "safe zone" of the radial head. The safe zone can be determined clinically by a subtended arc of 90°, with the arc midpoint directly lateral when the forearm is in the neutral position (Fig. 4) [61,62]. The safe zone can be visually confirmed because the cartilage is slightly grayish and thinner than the thicker, white cartilage of the articulating portion. Care should be taken to avoid screw tip penetration through the opposite cortex and to countersink the screw heads, particularly if the screws have been inserted outside the safe zone. Prominent internal fixation may interfere with forearm

rotation, irritate adjacent soft tissues, and require removal.

The role of arthroscopy remains undefined in the treatment of radial head fractures. The advantage of arthroscopy includes improved joint surface visualization without performing the usual releases associated with open surgery. A recent description of an arthroscopic technique for the percutaneous fixation of radial head fractures reported preliminary satisfactory functional outcomes [63].

Radial head excision

Radial head fractures that are displaced, too comminuted for stable anatomic internal fixation, and too large for fragment excision alone should

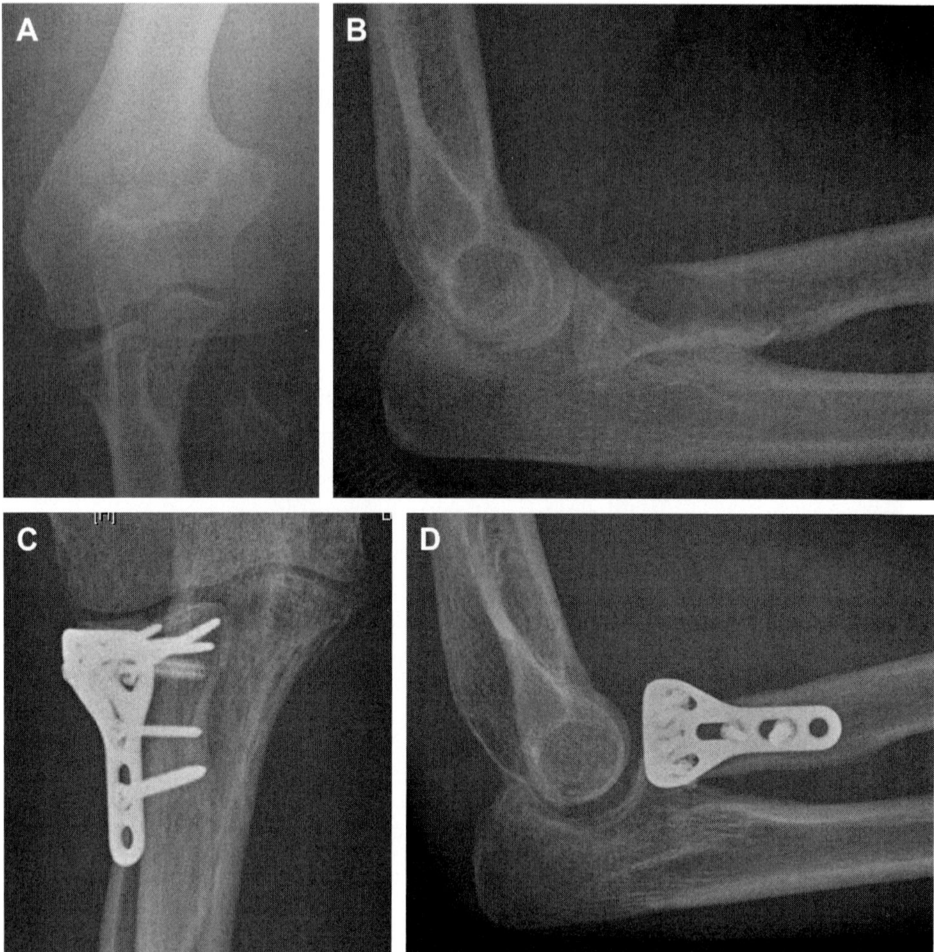

Fig. 3. Anteroposterior (*A*) and lateral (*B*) radiographs of a 26-year-old man who sustained a comminuted fracture of the radial head with metaphyseal extension. (*C*, *D*) Postoperative radiographs following ORIF of the radial head with a low profile radial head plate and fixed-angle locking screws. The patient developed a forearm rotation contracture requiring hardware removal and contracture release.

be managed by radial head excision with or without arthroplasty. Complete fragment excision can be confirmed with the use of an image intensifier and by reassembling all the fracture fragments.

Following excision of the radial head, elbow and forearm stability must be assessed clinically and fluoroscopically by varus/valgus and axial stress. The capitellum is evaluated for chondral injuries or osteochondral fractures. Associated fractures of the coronoid are managed as indicated, and their fixation should be performed before radial head replacement. In patients who have complex elbow instability, radial head excision without arthroplasty is contraindicated.

Resection of the radial head can be done arthroscopically (in cases in which radial head arthroplasty is not required) while providing the surgeon the ability to address other intra-articular pathologies [64,65].

Biomechanical data have demonstrated an alteration in the kinematics, load transfer, and stability of the elbow following radial head excision that may lead to premature cartilage wear of the ulnohumeral joint and to secondary pain due to arthritis [66,67]. Delayed radial head resection is intended to improve forearm rotation and to alleviate some of the pain originating from the radiocapitellar arthrosis in cases of radial head malunion or nonunion [41]. Long-term follow-up

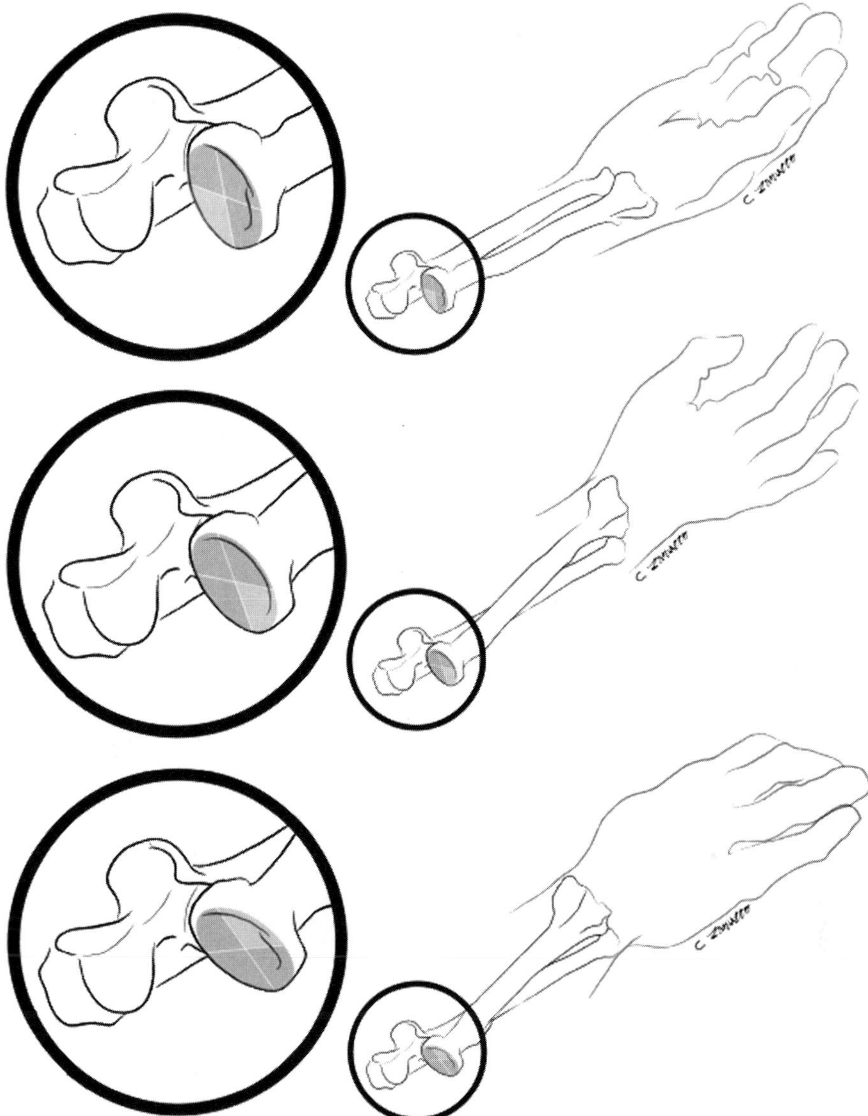

Fig. 4. The "safe zone" (*shaded in green*) for radial head plate application is demonstrated when the forearm is in supination, neutral, and pronation. (*Data from* Hotchkiss RN. Displaced fractures of the radial head: internal fixation or excision? J Am Acad Orthop Surg 1997;5(1):1–10.)

studies suggest a high incidence of radiographic arthritis with radial head excision, although the incidence of symptomatic arthritis varies widely among series [8–11,68,69].

Radial head arthroplasty

Radial head arthroplasty for fracture is indicated for unreconstructable displaced radial head fractures with an associated elbow dislocation or a known or possible disruption of the collateral or interosseous ligaments. Current available designs include monoblock metal implants [16,17], press-fit and ingrowth stems, cemented stems, bipolar implants [70], and ceramic designs. Various prosthetic materials have been employed for radial head arthroplasties, such as acrylic [71], silicone rubber [72], cobalt-chromium alloy [70,73], and titanium [16].

Silicone radial head arthroplasty, although initially successful in many patients, has been abandoned for several reasons [11,72,74,75]. First, silicone has been shown to provide little axial or valgus stability to the elbow, a feature that is critical in the setting of elbow instability [24]. Second, mechanical failure such as implant wear, fragmentation, and fracture was a frequent complication seen with this implant material. Third, synovitis due to particulate wear debris has been associated with progressive and generalized joint damage [76–79]. New modular metallic implants that closely match patient anatomy [80] and have simplified implantation have been developed to address the shortcomings of silicone radial head arthroplasty (Fig. 5A–D).

The resected radial head serves as a template for sizing of the prosthesis. At the time of trialing or implantation, the diameter, height, tracking, and congruency of the prosthesis is evaluated visually and with the aid of an image intensifier. The alignment of the distal radioulnar joint, ulnar variance, and the width of the lateral and medial portions of the ulnohumeral joint are checked under fluoroscopy. Overstuffing the radiocapitellar joint, suggested by a nonparallel medial ulnohumeral joint space that is wider laterally due to a radial head implant that is too thick, should be avoided to reduce the risk of cartilage wear on the capitellum from excessive pressure [81].

The short- and medium-term results of metallic radial head implants are encouraging. Moro and

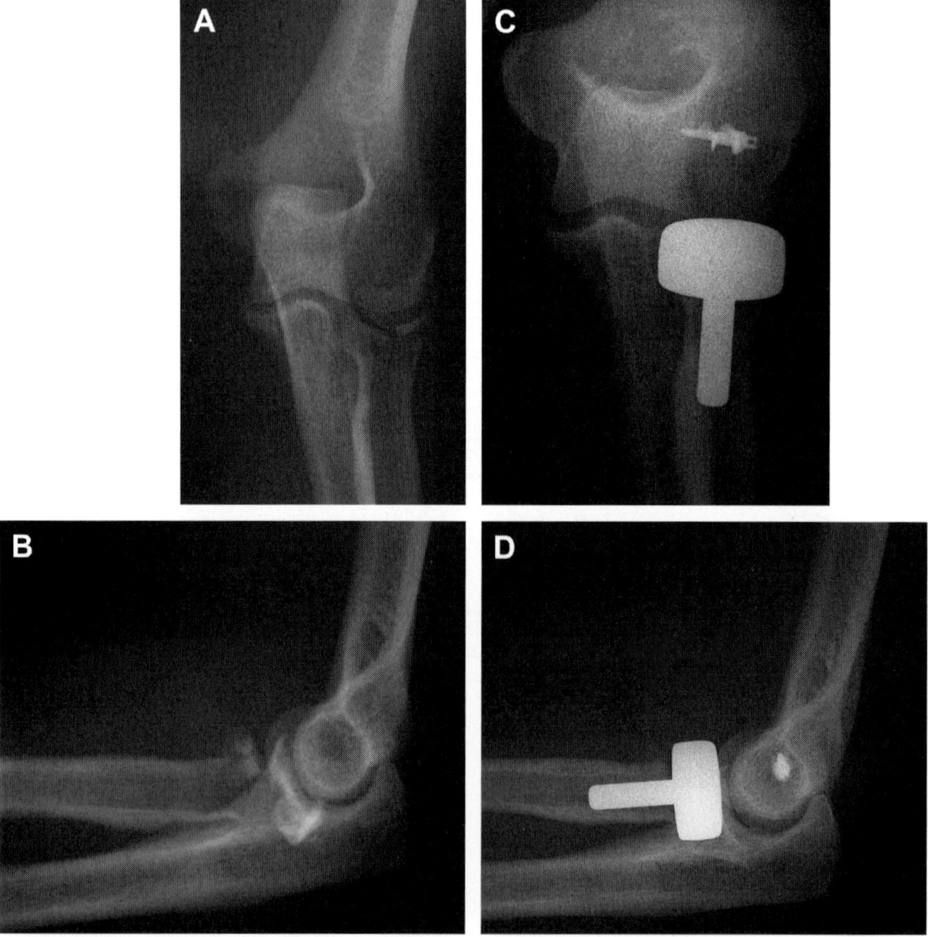

Fig. 5. Anteroposterior (*A*) and lateral (*B*) radiographs of a 47-year-old woman who sustained a comminuted radial head fracture to her left elbow. (*C*, *D*) The patient underwent modular radial head arthroplasty and repair of the lateral collateral ligaments using a suture anchor. Note that despite ligament repair, residual opening of the ulnohumeral joint is present on the immediate postoperative films (*D*).

colleagues [82] reported the functional outcome of 25 patients who had unreconstructable fractures of the radial head managed with a monoblock metallic radial head arthroplasty. The average follow-up was 39 months. The results were rated as good or excellent in 17 patients, fair in 5, and poor in 3, and no patient required removal of the implant. The radial head prosthesis was shown to restore elbow stability when stability was jeopardized; however, there were mild residual deficits in strength and motion. Grewal and colleagues [18] reported similar findings in a cohort of 26 patients treated with a modular metal radial head prosthesis.

Smets and colleagues [83] reported the results of a bipolar radial head prosthesis for comminuted acute Mason type III fractures of the radial head in 13 patients. The mean follow-up was 25 months. The results were rated as excellent or good in 10 patients and fair or poor in 3 patients, and one prosthesis was removed after 8 months due to severely decreased elbow function. There were no dislocations, hardware failures, or signs of loosening, even though the polyethylene insert has the potential to create wear debris leading to osteolysis and loosening. Dotzis and colleagues [20] reported the medium-term results of the Judet floating radial head prosthesis for comminuted radial head fractures in 12 patients at a mean follow up of 5.25 years. There were 10 excellent and good results, 1 fair, and 1 poor, with one significant complication of complex regional pain syndrome. There was no evidence of secondary elbow instability, implant loosening, or osteoporosis of the capitellum.

There is a paucity of literature reporting the long-term outcomes of radial head arthroplasty with respect to loosening, capitellar wear, and arthritis. Harrington and colleagues [17] reported their experience with metallic radial head arthroplasty in 20 patients at an average follow-up of 12 years. The results were excellent or good in 16 patients and fair or poor in 4. Metallic radial head replacement has been shown to provide good clinical and radiographic outcomes in most patients at short- and medium-term follow-up, but additional long-term outcome studies are necessary.

Lateral ligament complex repair

The lateral ligament complex is an important stabilizer against varus and posterolateral rotational instability of the elbow. Following radial head repair or replacement, the lateral ligament complex and extensor muscle origins are repaired to the lateral epicondyle. If the lateral ulnar collateral ligament (posterior portion of lateral ligment complex) remains attached to the lateral epicondyle, then the anterior half of the lateral ligament complex (the annular ligament and radial collateral ligament) is repaired to the posterior half. This repair is followed by closure of the muscle-splitting interval that was used for initial exposure.

The lateral collateral ligament and the extensor origin should be securely repaired to the lateral epicondyle if they have been completely detached by the injury or by surgical exposure. Nonabsorbable running locked sutures grasp the ligament and are passed through diverging transosseous tunnels that originate from the center of rotation of the radiocapitellar joint (the center of the arc of curvature of the capitellum), which is the origin of the lateral ulnar collateral ligament. Suture anchors inserted into the center of rotation of the radiocapitellar joint can also be used for ligament repair. A disadvantage of suture anchors is that in cases of complex elbow instability requiring hinged external fixation (acutely or for delay chronic instability requiring reconstruction), insertion of the fixator center axis pin can be blocked by the previously placed suture anchor. For this reason and for cost saving, the authors prefer the transosseous repair technique. After the ligament has been repaired, the capsule is closed and the common extensor origin is repaired to the lateral supracondylar ridge.

Following ORIF or arthroplasty and lateral soft tissue repair, the elbow should be placed through an arc of flexion-extension to carefully evaluate for elbow stability in pronation, neutral, and supination [84,85]. Patients who have persistent instability may require repair of the medial collateral ligament and flexor pronator origin if the elbow subluxates at 40° or more of flexion.

Rehabilitation

For an isolated radial head replacement treated with a lateral ulnar collateral ligament sparing approach, active ROM should be initiated on the day following surgery. A collar and cuff with the elbow maintained at 90° is employed for comfort between exercises. A static progressive extension splint is fabricated for nighttime use for patients who do not have associated ligamentous disruptions and is employed for a period of

12 weeks. The splint is adjusted weekly as extension improves. In patients who have associated elbow dislocations or residual instability, extension splinting is not implemented until 6 weeks after surgery.

Patients who have associated fractures, dislocations, or ligamentous injuries should commence active flexion and extension motion within a safe arc 1 day postoperatively. Active forearm rotation is performed with the elbow in flexion to minimize stress on the medial or lateral ligamentous injuries or repairs. Extension is performed with the forearm in the appropriate rotational position, that is, pronation, if the lateral ligaments are deficient and the medial ligaments are intact [49]; supination, if the medial ligaments are deficient and the lateral ligaments are intact/repaired [86]; and neutral, if both sides have been injured/repaired. A resting splint with the elbow maintained at 90° and the forearm in the appropriate rotation is employed for 3 to 6 weeks. Passive stretching is not permitted for 6 weeks to reduce the incidence of repair attenuation and heterotopic ossification. Strengthening exercises are initiated after the ligament injuries and any associated fractures have adequately healed, usually at 8 to 12 weeks postoperatively.

For patients who have complex elbow injury undergoing any surgical intervention on the radial head, prophylactic therapy with oral indomethacin, 25 mg three times a day for 3 weeks, may be considered to potentially lower the incidence of heterotopic ossification.

Complications

Posterior interosseous nerve injury can occur as a consequence of dissection distal to the radial tuberosity or due to placement of anterior retractors around the radial neck [46]. A recent study showed that the posterior interosseous nerve is an average of 3.8 cm distal to the articular surface of the radius during pronation [47]. The forearm should be pronated while exposing the radial head, especially when the EDC splitting approach is being used. Some investigators recommend identifying the nerve when dissection onto the radial neck is required [35].

Stiffness, nonunion, malunion, avascular necrosis, and painful/prominent hardware are complications associated with radial head fractures [15,32,50,87]. Stiffness is the most frequent complication and can be due to capsular contracture, scarring of the annular ligament, heterotopic ossification, or retained cartilaginous or osseous fragments. In cases of stiffness due to capsular contracture, passive stretching should be initiated under the supervision of a physical therapist, with the concomitant use of static progressive splints. A flexion cuff may be used to regain terminal elbow flexion [87]. In refractory cases, turnbuckle splinting should be instituted 12 to 16 weeks postoperatively [88], and dynamic prosupination splinting should be used in cases of reduced forearm rotation [89]. In recalcitrant cases, open or arthroscopic capsular release may be done with satisfactory outcomes [87,90].

Instability or recurrent dislocations of the elbow due to an inadequate or failed ligament repair can be addressed with protective splinting, ligament reconstruction, or application of an articulated external fixator.

Prosthetic loosening, polyethelene wear, and capitellar wear and pain due to an overstuffed implant are complications associated with radial head arthroplasty [81,91]. Post-traumatic arthritis of the capitellum may arise due to articular cartilage damage from the initial injury or from persistent instability or may be due to increased loads transmitted to the capitellum from an overstuffed radial head arthroplasty. If the radial head implant requires removal for any reason, then the elbow must be carefully examined to ensure valgus and axial stability.

Summary

Radial head fractures are the most common elbow fracture. Nevertheless, there is a paucity of literature demonstrating the long-term results of internal fixation of displaced radial head fractures and of radial head arthroplasty. Consensus exists in the literature regarding the nonsurgical treatment of undisplaced radial head fractures. Controversy surrounds the indications for surgery and the most appropriate intervention for displaced fractures. Further research is necessary to provide a better scientific rationale for making treatment recommendations. There is a need for better guidelines as to which radial head fractures should be treated nonoperatively, which should be managed surgically with ORIF, and which should be treated with a radial head excision with or without arthroplasty.

References

[1] Davidson PA, Moseley JB Jr, Tullos HS. Radial head fracture. A potentially complex injury. Clin Orthop Relat Res 1993;297:224–30.

[2] Ring D, Jupiter JB, Zilberfarb J. Posterior dislocation of the elbow with fractures of the radial head and coronoid. J Bone Joint Surg Am 2002;84(4): 547–51.

[3] Dubberley JH, Faber KJ, Macdermid JC, et al. Outcome after open reduction and internal fixation of capitellar and trochlear fractures. J Bone Joint Surg Am 2006;88(1):46–54.

[4] Struijs PA, Smit G, Steller EP. Radial head fractures: effectiveness of conservative treatment versus surgical intervention: a systematic review. Arch Orthop Trauma Surg 2007;127(2):125–30.

[5] Van Glabbeek F, Van Riet R, Verstreken J. Current concepts in the treatment of radial head fractures in the adult. A clinical and biomechanical approach. Acta Orthop Belg 2001;67(5):430–41.

[6] Radin EL, Riseborough EJ. Fractures of the radial head. A review of eighty-eight cases and analysis of the indications for excision of the radial head and non-operative treatment. J Bone Joint Surg Am 1966;48(6):1055–64.

[7] Carstam N. Operative treatment of fractures of the head and neck of the radius. Acta Orthop Scand 1950;19(4):502–26.

[8] Ikeda M, Oka Y. Function after early radial head resection for fracture: a retrospective evaluation of 15 patients followed for 3–18 years. Acta Orthop Scand 2000;71(2):191–4.

[9] Janssen RP, Vegter J. Resection of the radial head after Mason type-III fractures of the elbow: follow-up at 16 to 30 years. J Bone Joint Surg Br 1998;80(2):231–3.

[10] Goldberg I, Peylan J, Yosipovitch Z. Late results of excision of the radial head for an isolated closed fracture. J Bone Joint Surg Am 1986;68(5):675–9.

[11] Boulas HJ, Morrey BF. Biomechanical evaluation of the elbow following radial head fracture. Comparison of open reduction and internal fixation vs. excision, Silastic replacement, and non-operative management. Chir Main 1998;17(4):314–20.

[12] Esser RD, Davis S, Taavao T. Fractures of the radial head treated by internal fixation: late results in 26 cases. J Orthop Trauma 1995;9(4):318–23.

[13] Odenheimer K, Harvey JP Jr. Internal fixation of fracture of the head of the radius. Two case reports. J Bone Joint Surg Am 1979;61(5):785–7.

[14] Khalfayan EE, Culp RW, Alexander AH. Mason type II radial head fractures: operative versus nonoperative treatment. J Orthop Trauma 1992; 6(3):283–9.

[15] King GJ, Evans DC, Kellam JF. Open reduction and internal fixation of radial head fractures. J Orthop Trauma 1991;5(1):21–8.

[16] Harrington IJ, Tountas AA. Replacement of the radial head in the treatment of unstable elbow fractures. Injury 1981;12(5):405–12.

[17] Harrington IJ, Sekyi-Otu A, Barrington TW, et al. The functional outcome with metallic radial head implants in the treatment of unstable elbow fractures: a long-term review. J Trauma 2001;50(1): 46–52.

[18] Grewal R, MacDermid JC, Faber KJ, et al. Comminuted radial head fractures treated with a modular metallic radial head arthroplasty. Study of outcomes. J Bone Joint Surg Am 2006;88(10):2192–200.

[19] Frosch KH, Knopp W, Dresing K, et al. A bipolar radial head prosthesis after comminuted radial head fractures: indications, treatment and outcome after 5 years). Unfallchirurg 2003;106(5):367–73 [in German].

[20] Dotzis A, Cochu G, Mabit C, et al. Comminuted fractures of the radial head treated by the Judet floating radial head prosthesis. J Bone Joint Surg Br 2006;88(6):760–4.

[21] Chapman CB, Su BW, Sinicropi SM, et al. Vitallium radial head prosthesis for acute and chronic elbow fractures and fracture-dislocations involving the radial head. J Shoulder Elbow Surg 2006;15(4):463–73.

[22] Cugola L, Vecchini L. [Use of a Silastic prosthesis in traumatic and degenerative lesions of the radial head]. Clin Ortop 1974;25(1):11–6 [in Italian].

[23] Pomianowski S, Morrey BF, Neale PG, et al. Contribution of monoblock and bipolar radial head prostheses to valgus stability of the elbow. J Bone Joint Surg Am 2001;83(12):1829–34.

[24] King GJ, Zarzour ZD, Rath DA, et al. Metallic radial head arthroplasty improves valgus stability of the elbow. Clin Orthop Relat Res 1999;368:114–25.

[25] Morrey BF, An KN. Articular and ligamentous contributions to the stability of the elbow joint. Am J Sports Med 1983;11(5):315–9.

[26] Morrey BF, Tanaka S, An KN. Valgus stability of the elbow. A definition of primary and secondary constraints. Clin Orthop Relat Res 1991;265: 187–95.

[27] O'Driscoll SW, Bell DF, Morrey BF. Posterolateral rotatory instability of the elbow. J Bone Joint Surg Am 1991;73(3):440–6.

[28] Beingessner DM, Dunning CE, Gordon KD, et al. The effect of radial head fracture size on elbow kinematics and stability. J Orthop Res 2005;23(1):210–7.

[29] Halls AA, Travill A. Transmission of pressures across the elbow joint. Anat Rec 1964;150:243–7.

[30] Essex-Lopresti P. Fractures of the radial head with distal radioulnar dislocation. J Bone Joint Surg Br 1951;33:244–7.

[31] Ring D, Jupiter JB. Current concepts review: fracture-dislocation of the elbow. J Bone Joint Surg Am 1998;80(4):566–80.

[32] Mason ML. Some observations on fractures of the head of the radius with a review of one hundred cases. Br J Surg 1954;42(172):123–32.

[33] Johnston GW. A follow-up of one hundred cases of fracture of the head of the radius with a review of the literature. Ulster Med J 1962;31:51–6.

[34] Morrey BF. Radial head fractures. In: The elbow and its disorders. Philadelphia: WB Saunders; 1985. p. 355–81.

[35] Hotchkiss RN. Displaced fractures of the radial head: internal fixation or excision? J Am Acad Orthop Surg 1997;5(1):1–10.

[36] Morgan SJ, Groshen SL, Itamura JM, et al. Reliability evaluation of classifying radial head fractures by the system of Mason. Bull Hosp Jt Dis 1997;56(2):95–8.

[37] Liow RY, Cregan A, Nanda R, et al. Early mobilisation for minimally displaced radial head fractures is desirable. A prospective randomised study of two protocols. Injury 2002;33(9):801–6.

[38] Holdsworth BJ, Clement DA, Rothwell PN. Fractures of the radial head—the benefit of aspiration: a prospective controlled trial. Injury 1987;18(1):44–7.

[39] Betz A. [Surgical differential therapy of fracture of the radius head]. Orthopade 1988;17(3):320–7 [in German].

[40] Weseley MS, Barenfeld PA, Eisenstein AL. Closed treatment of isolated radial head fractures. J Trauma 1983;23(1):36–9.

[41] Broberg MA, Morrey BF. Results of delayed excision of the radial head after fracture. J Bone Joint Surg Am 1986;68(5):669–74.

[42] Akesson T, Herbertsson P, Josefsson PO, et al. Primary nonoperative treatment of moderately displaced two-part fractures of the radial head. J Bone Joint Surg Am 2006;88(9):1909–14.

[43] Dowdy PA, Bain GI, King GJ, et al. The midline posterior elbow incision. An anatomical appraisal. J Bone Joint Surg Br 1995;77(5):696–9.

[44] Patterson SD, Bain GI, Mehta JA. Surgical approaches to the elbow. Clin Orthop Relat Res 2000;370:19–33.

[45] McKee MD, Pugh DMW, Wild LM, et al. Standard surgical protocol to treat elbow dislocations with radial head and coronoid fractures. Surgical technique. J Bone Joint Surg Am 2005;87(Suppl 1 Pt 1):22–32.

[46] Strachan JC, Ellis BW. Vulnerability of the posterior interosseous nerve during radial head resection. J Bone Joint Surg Br 1971;53(2):320–3.

[47] Diliberti T, Botte MJ, Abrams RA. Anatomical considerations regarding the posterior interosseous nerve during posterolateral approaches to the proximal part of the radius. J Bone Joint Surg Am 2000; 82(6):809–13.

[48] Kocher T. Textbook of operative surgery. 3rd edition. London: Adam and Charles Black; 1911.

[49] Dunning CE, Zarzour ZD, Patterson SD, et al. Ligamentous stabilizers against posterolateral rotatory instability of the elbow. J Bone Joint Surg Am 2001;83-A(12):1823–8.

[50] Ring D, Quintero J, Jupiter JB. Open reduction and internal fixation of fractures of the radial head. J Bone Joint Surg Am 2002;84(10):1811–5.

[51] Ikeda M, Sugiyama K, Kang C, et al. Comminuted fractures of the radial head. Comparison of resection and internal fixation. J Bone Joint Surg Am 2005; 87(1):76–84.

[52] Ikeda M, Yamashina Y, Kamimoto M, et al. Open reduction and internal fixation of comminuted fractures of the radial head using low-profile miniplates. J Bone Joint Surg Br 2003;85(7):1040–4.

[53] Bunker TD, Newman JH. The Herbert differential pitch bone screw in displaced radial head fractures. Injury 1985;16(9):621–4.

[54] Pearce MS, Gallannaugh SC. Mason type II radial head fractures fixed with Herbert bone screws. J R Soc Med 1996;89(6):340P–4P.

[55] Arcalis Arce A, Marti Garin D, Molero Garcia V, et al. Treatment of radial head fractures using a fibrin adhesive seal. A review of 15 cases. J Bone Joint Surg Br 1995;77(3):422–4.

[56] Hirvensalo E, Bostman O, Rokkanen P. Absorbable polyglycolide pins in fixation of displaced fractures of the radial head. Arch Orthop Trauma Surg 1990;109(5):258–61.

[57] Pelto K, Hirvensalo E, Bostman O, et al. Treatment of radial head fractures with absorbable polyglycolide pins: a study on the security of the fixation in 38 cases. J Orthop Trauma 1994;8(2): 94–8.

[58] Prokop A, Jubel A, Helling HJ, et al. [New biodegradable polylactide implants (Polypin-C) in therapy for radial head fractures]. Chirurg 2002;73(10): 997–1004 [in German].

[59] Helling HJ, Prokop A, Schmid HU, et al. Biodegradable implants versus standard metal fixation for displaced radial head fractures. A prospective, randomized, multicenter study. J Shoulder Elbow Surg 2006;15(4):479–85.

[60] Giffin JR, King GJ, Patterson SD, et al. Internal fixation of radial neck fractures: an in vitro biomechanical analysis. Clin Biomech (Bristol, Avon) 2004;19(4):358–61.

[61] Smith GR, Hotchkiss RN. Radial head and neck fractures: anatomic guidelines for proper placement of internal fixation. J Shoulder Elbow Surg 1996; 5(2 Pt 1):113–7.

[62] Soyer AD, Nowotarski PJ, Kelso TB, et al. Optimal position for plate fixation of complex fractures of the proximal radius: a cadaver study. J Orthop Trauma 1998;12(4):291–3.

[63] Rolla PR, Surace MF, Bini A, et al. Arthroscopic treatment of fractures of the radial head. Arthroscopy 2006;22(2):233.e1–6.

[64] Menth-Chiari WA, Ruch DS, Poehling GG. Arthroscopic excision of the radial head: clinical outcome in 12 patients with post-traumatic arthritis after fracture of the radial head or rheumatoid arthritis. Arthroscopy 2001;17(9):918–23.

[65] Lo IK, King GJ. Arthroscopic radial head excision. Arthroscopy 1994;10(6):689–92.

[66] Beingessner DM, Dunning CE, Gordon KD, et al. The effect of radial head excision and arthroplasty on elbow kinematics and stability. J Bone Joint Surg Am 2004;86(8):1730–9.

[67] Jensen SL, Olsen BS, Sojbjerg JO. Elbow joint kinematics after excision of the radial head. J Shoulder Elbow Surg 1999;8(3):238–41.

[68] Coleman DA, Blair WF, Shurr D. Resection of the radial head for fracture of the radial head. Long-term follow-up of seventeen cases. J Bone Joint Surg Am 1987;69(3):385–92.

[69] Mikic ZD, Vukadinovic SM. Late results in fractures of the radial head treated by excision. Clin Orthop Relat Res 1983;181:220–8.

[70] Judet T, Garreau de Loubresse C, Piriou P, et al. A floating prosthesis for radial-head fractures. J Bone Joint Surg Br 1996;78(2):244–9.

[71] Cherry JC. Use of acrylic prosthesis in the treatment of fracture of the head of the radius. J Bone Joint Surg Br 1953;35(1):70–1.

[72] Swanson AB, Jaeger SH, La Rochelle D. Comminuted fractures of the radial head. The role of silicone-implant replacement arthroplasty. J Bone Joint Surg Am 1981;63(7):1039–49.

[73] Knight DJ, Rymaszewski LA, Amis AA, et al. Primary replacement of the fractured radial head with a metal prosthesis. J Bone Joint Surg Br 1993; 75(4):572–6.

[74] Berger M, Urvoy P, Mestdagh H. [A comparative study of the treatment of fractures of the radial head by resection or by Swanson Silastic implant]. Ann Radiol (Paris) 1991;34(5):330–7 [in French].

[75] Carn RM, Medige J, Curtain D, et al. Silicone rubber replacement of the severely fractured radial head. Clin Orthop Relat Res 1986;209:259–69.

[76] Gordon M, Bullough PG. Synovial and osseous inflammation in failed silicone-rubber prostheses. J Bone Joint Surg Am 1982;64(4):574–80.

[77] Mayhall WS, Tiley FT, Paluska DJ. Fracture of Silastic radial-head prosthesis. Case report. J Bone Joint Surg Am 1981;63(3):459–60.

[78] Stoffelen DV, Holdsworth BJ. Excision or Silastic replacement for comminuted radial head fractures. A long-term follow-up. Acta Orthop Belg 1994; 60(4):402–7.

[79] Vanderwilde RS, Morrey BF, Melberg MW, et al. Inflammatory arthritis after failure of silicone rubber replacement of the radial head. J Bone Joint Surg Br 1994;76(1):78–81.

[80] King GJ, Zarzour ZD, Patterson SD, et al. An anthropometric study of the radial head: implications in the design of a prosthesis. J Arthroplasty 2001;16(1):112–6.

[81] Van Riet RP, Van Glabbeek F, Verborgt O, et al. Capitellar erosion caused by a metal radial head prosthesis. A case report. J Bone Joint Surg Am 2004;86-A(5):1061–4.

[82] Moro JK, Werier J, MacDermid JC, et al. Arthroplasty with a metal radial head for unreconstructible fractures of the radial head. J Bone Joint Surg Am 2001;83(8):1201–11.

[83] Smets S, Govaers K, Jansen N, et al. The floating radial head prosthesis for comminuted radial head fractures: a multicentric study. Acta Orthop Belg 2000;66(4):353–8.

[84] Bain GI, Ashwood N, Baird R, et al. Management of Mason type-III radial head fractures with a titanium prosthesis, ligament repair, and early mobilization. Surgical technique. J Bone Joint Surg Am 2005; 87(Suppl 1 Pt 1):136–47.

[85] Hildebrand KA, Patterson SD, King GJ. Acute elbow dislocations: simple and complex. Orthop Clin North Am 1999;30(1):63–79.

[86] Armstrong AD, Dunning CE, Faber KJ, et al. Rehabilitation of the medial collateral ligament-deficient elbow: an in vitro biomechanical study. J Hand Surg [Am] 2000;25(6):1051–7.

[87] King GJ, Faber KJ. Posttraumatic elbow stiffness. Orthop Clin North Am 2000;31(1):129–43.

[88] Gelinas JJ, Faber KJ, Patterson SD, et al. The effectiveness of turnbuckle splinting for elbow contractures. J Bone Joint Surg Br 2000;82(1):74–8.

[89] Shah MA, Lopez JK, Escalante AS, et al. Dynamic splinting of forearm rotational contracture after distal radius fracture. J Hand Surg [Am] 2002; 27(3):456–63.

[90] Nguyen D, Proper SI, MacDermid JC, et al. Functional outcomes of arthroscopic capsular release of the elbow. Arthroscopy 2006;22(8):842–9.

[91] van Riet RP, Van Glabbeek F, Baumfeld JA, et al. The effect of the orientation of the radial head on the kinematics of the ulnohumeral joint and force transmission through the radiocapitellar joint. Clin Biomech (Bristol, Avon) 2006;21(6): 554–9.

satisfied with their outcome. The flexion and extension peak torque losses observed in this study were consistent with other studies [22,49,52].

Aslam and Willett [70] also reported on the functional outcome of 26 patients (all older than 60 years of age) who had AO type C fractures treated with orthogonal plating. Good to excellent results were achieved in 70% of patients who had a mean flexion/extension arc of 112 degrees. Grip strength was 82% compared with the uninjured side. Hardware removal was required in 15% of the cases and the overall complication rate was 35%, which is consistent with other studies [48,66]. Eighty-five percent of patients were satisfied with their final outcome and 75% of patients returned to their preinjury level of occupation and activity [70].

Nonunion

The average time to union of distal humerus fractures has been reported to be 14.6 weeks [6]. Nonunion of distal humerus fractures treated with ORIF has been reported to be between 2% and 10% [71]. In the Helfet and colleagues [71] series of 33 distal humerus nonunions, 75% were the result of failed internal fixation. A 98% union rate was obtained following revision ORIF. A total of 29% of patients needed additional surgery after the revision procedure and complications included two superficial infections, two deep infections, and five cases of ulnar neuropathy. Based on this study, the authors concluded that successful treatment of distal humeral nonunions requires aggressive contracture release, stable fixation, and autogenous bone graft [18,71].

Heterotropic ossification

The reported incidence of heterotropic ossification (HO) after surgical treatment of distal humerus fractures varies from 0% [6,38] to 49% [15]. In most patients, HO does not cause functional deficits [10,13,22] and resection is not always necessary [8]. Some studies have found that a delay in treatment of greater than 48 hours increases the rate of HO from 0% to 33% [41,72]. Similarly, Kundel and colleagues [15] reported an increased rate of HO from 29% to 80% when surgical treatment was delayed by more than 24 hours, which was also associated with significantly worse ROM and function. The routine use of indomethacin for HO prophylaxis remains controversial.

Summary

Intra-articular fractures of the distal humerus are among the most challenging fractures to manage. Nonoperative treatment, although appropriate for some patients, often leads to loss of motion and unsatisfactory functional outcomes. Over the last 2 decades, enhanced operative techniques and implant designs have improved the reduction and stability of distal humerus fractures leading to better outcomes. Careful preoperative planning, adequate exposure, and stable fixation facilitating early mobilization are essential to achieve successful outcomes with internal fixation.

References

[1] Riseborough EJ, Radin EL. Intercondylar T fractures of the humerus in the adult. A comparison of operative and non-operative treatment in twenty-nine cases. J Bone Joint Surg Am 1969;51:130–41.

[2] O'Driscoll SW. Supracondylar fractures of the elbow: open reduction, internal fixation [review]. Hand Clin 2004;20:465–74.

[3] Ring D, Jupiter JB. Complex fractures of the distal humerus and their complications [review]. J Shoulder Elbow Surg 1999;8:85–97.

[4] Korner J, Lill H, Muller LP, et al. Distal humerus fractures in elderly patients: results after open reduction and internal fixation. Osteoporos Int 2005; 16(Suppl 2):S73–9.

[5] O'Driscoll SW. Optimizing stability in distal humeral fracture fixation. J Shoulder Elbow Surg 2005;14:186S–194S.

[6] Huang TL, Chiu FY, Chuang TY, et al. The results of open reduction and internal fixation in elderly patients with severe fractures of the distal humerus: a critical analysis of the results. J Trauma 2005;58:62–9.

[7] Allende CA, Allende BT, Allende BL, et al. Intercondylar distal humerus fractures—surgical treatment and results. Chir Main 2004;23:85–95.

[8] Tyllianakis M, Panagopoulos A, Papadopoulos AX, et al. Functional evaluation of comminuted intra-articular fractures of the distal humerus (AO type C). Long term results in twenty-six patients. Acta Orthop Belg 2004;70:123–30.

[9] Soon JL, Chan BK, Low CO. Surgical fixation of intra-articular fractures of the distal humerus in adults [see comment] [erratum appears in Injury. 2004 Sep;35(9):954]. Injury 2004;35:44–54.

[10] Gupta R, Khanchandani P. Intercondylar fractures of the distal humerus in adults: a critical analysis of 55 cases. Injury 2002;33:511–5.

[11] O'Driscoll SW, Sanchez-Sotelo J, Torchia ME. Management of the smashed distal humerus [review]. Orthop Clin North Am 2002;33:19–33.

[12] Ring D, Jupiter JB. Fractures of the distal humerus [review]. Orthop Clin North Am 2000;31:103–13.

[13] Kinik H, Atalar H, Mergen E. Management of distal humerus fractures in adults. Arch Orthop Trauma Surg 1999;119:467–9.

[14] Gupta R. Intercondylar fractures of the distal humerus in adults. Injury 1996;27:569–72.

[15] Kundel K, Braun W, Wieberneit J, et al. Intraarticular distal humerus fractures. Factors affecting functional outcome. Clin Orthop Relat Res 1996;332:200–8.

[16] Papaioannou N, Babis GC, Kalavritinos J, et al. Operative treatment of type C intra-articular fractures of the distal humerus: the role of stability achieved at surgery on final outcome. Injury 1995; 26:169–73.

[17] McKee MD, Jupiter JB. A contemporary approach to the management of complex fractures of the distal humerus and their sequelae [review]. Hand Clin 1994;10:479–94.

[18] Helfet DL, Schmeling GJ. Bicondylar intraarticular fractures of the distal humerus in adults [review]. Clin Orthop Relat Res 1993;292:26–36.

[19] Sanders RA, Raney EM, Pipkin S. Operative treatment of bicondylar intraarticular fractures of the distal humerus. Orthopedics 1992;15:159–63.

[20] Gabel GT, Hanson G, Bennett JB, et al. Intraarticular fractures of the distal humerus in the adult. Clin Orthop Relat Res 1987;216:99–108.

[21] Horne G. Supracondylar fractures of the humerus in adults. J Trauma 1980;20:71–4.

[22] Gofton WT, Macdermid JC, Patterson SD, et al. Functional outcome of AO type C distal humeral fractures. J Hand Surg [Am] 2003;28:294–308.

[23] Pajarinen J, Bjorkenheim JM. Operative treatment of type C intercondylar fractures of the distal humerus: results after a mean follow-up of 2 years in a series of 18 patients. J Shoulder Elbow Surg 2002;11:48–52.

[24] Ruedi T, Buckley R, Moran C. AO principles of fracture managment. 2nd expanded edition. New York: Thieme Medical Publishing; 2007.

[25] Anglen J. Distal humerus fractures [review]. J Am Acad Orthop Surg 2005;13:291–7.

[26] Palvanen M, Kannus P, Niemi S, et al. Secular trends in the osteoporotic fractures of the distal humerus in elderly women. Eur J Epidemiol 1998; 14:159–64.

[27] Palvanen M, Kannus P, Parkkari J, et al. The injury mechanisms of osteoporotic upper extremity fractures among older adults: a controlled study of 287 consecutive patients and their 108 controls. Osteoporos Int 2000;11:822–31.

[28] Robinson CM, Hill RM, Jacobs N, et al. Adult distal humeral metaphyseal fractures: epidemiology and results of treatment [see comment]. J Orthop Trauma 2003;17:38–47.

[29] McCarty LP, Ring D, Jupiter JB. Management of distal humerus fractures [review]. Am J Orthop 2005;34:430–8.

[30] Jupiter JB, Mehne DK. Fractures of the distal humerus [review]. Orthopedics 1992;15:825–33.

[31] Ring D, Jupiter JB. Elbow and forearm: adult trauma. In: Vaccaro A, editor. Orthopaedic knowledge update 8. Rosemont (IL): AAOS; 2005. p. 307–15.

[32] Muller M, Nazanan S, Koch P, et al. Fracture and dislocation compendium. Orthopaedic trauma association committee for coding and classification. J Orthop Trauma 2001;10(Suppl 1):311–24.

[33] Lowden C, Garvin G, King GJ. Imaging of the elbow following trauma [review]. Hand Clin 2004; 20:353–61.

[34] Eastwood W. The T-shaped fracture of the lower end of the humerus. J Bone Joint Surg Am 1937; 19:364–9.

[35] Dowdy PA, Bain GI, King GJ, et al. The midline posterior elbow incision. An anatomical appraisal. J Bone Joint Surg Br 1995;77:696–9.

[36] Athwal GS, Rispoli DM, Steinmann SP. The anconeus flap transolecranon approach to the distal humerus. J Orthop Trauma 2006;20:282–5.

[37] Wilkinson JM, Stanley D. Posterior surgical approaches to the elbow: a comparative anatomic study [see comment]. J Shoulder Elbow Surg 2001; 10:380–2.

[38] Eralp L, Kocaoglu M, Sar C, et al. Surgical treatment of distal intraarticular humeral fractures in adults. Int Orthop 2001;25:46–50.

[39] Wang KC, Shih HN, Hsu KY, et al. Intercondylar fractures of the distal humerus: routine anterior subcutaneous transposition of the ulnar nerve in a posterior operative approach. J Trauma 1994;36:770–3.

[40] Gainor BJ, Moussa F, Schott T. Healing rate of transverse osteotomies of the olecranon used in reconstruction of distal humerus fractures. J South Orthop Assoc 1995;4:263–8.

[41] Holdsworth BJ, Mossad MM. Fractures of the adult distal humerus. Elbow function after internal fixation. J Bone Joint Surg Br 1990;72:362–5.

[42] Hewins EA, Gofton WT, Dubberly J, et al. Plate fixation of olecranon osteotomies. J Orthop Trauma 2007;21:58–62.

[43] Coles CP, Barei DP, Nork SE, et al. The olecranon osteotomy: a six-year experience in the treatment of intraarticular fractures of the distal humerus. J Orthop Trauma 2006;20:164–71.

[44] Ring D, Gulotta L, Chin K, et al. Olecranon osteotomy for exposure of fractures and nonunions of the distal humerus. J Orthop Trauma 2004;18:446–9.

[45] Alonso-Llames M. Bilaterotricipital approach to the elbow. Its application in the osteosynthesis of supracondylar fractures of the humerus in children. Acta Orthop Scand 1972;43:479–90.

[46] Schildhauer TA, Nork SE, Mills WJ, et al. Extensor mechanism-sparing paratricipital posterior approach to the distal humerus. J Orthop Trauma 2003;17: 374–8.

[47] Campbell WC. Incision for exposure of the elbow joint. Am J Surg 1932;15:65–7.

[48] McKee MD, Kim J, Kebaish K, et al. Functional outcome after open supracondylar fractures of the

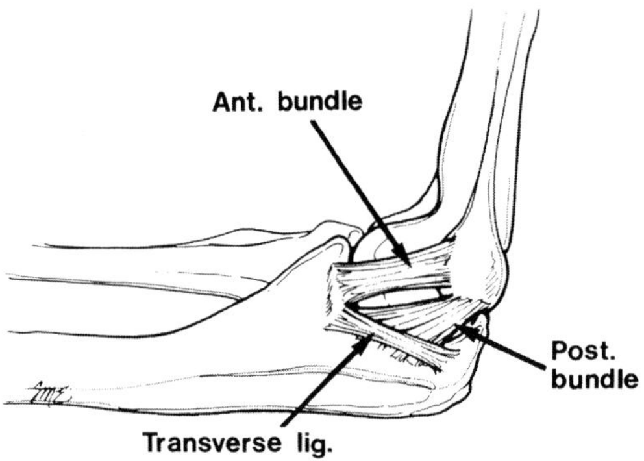

Fig. 1. Anatomy of the medial ulnar collateral ligament of the elbow showing anterior, posterior, and transverse bundles.

anterior bundle is the primary restraint to valgus stress at 30°, 60°, and 90°. The anterior and posterior bundles share the primary load at 120° of flexion [3]. The remaining varus torque needed is produced by the radiocapitellar joint and the flexor/pronator mass. It should be noted that forearm rotation has a large effect on the tension of the static and dynamic structures of the medial elbow, with maximum pronation giving the most laxity [10].

Mechanism of injury

Most medial instability patterns are found in throwing athletes over an extended period of time. Most athletes are unable to recall a specific event leading to instability but instead develop instability progressively over time as a result of repetitive microtrauma. The medial ulnar collateral ligament stretches or tears because of the valgus stress it must absorb during throwing motion. Occasionally, athletes recall one inciting throw in which a "pop" was felt or heard, which indicates an acute tear of the medial ulnar collateral ligament. The resulting instability with medial ulnar collateral ligament insufficiency becomes apparent with pain medially during the late cocking and acceleration phases and can be accompanied by complaints of loss of control and velocity early in the course. Rarely, a nonthrower continues to have chronic, persistent medial instability that causes difficulty in industrial-type labor. Bennett and colleagues [11] reported on a series of 14 such patients who required reconstructive surgery for chronic medial elbow instability, with 13 of the patients achieving good to excellent results.

Clinical examination

A thorough examination of the affected upper extremity begins with assessment of neurovascular status with careful attention to the ulnar nerve. The elbow must be assessed for carrying angle, range of motion to include flexion contracture, and pronation/supination arc of motion. The function of the flexor/pronator mass should be tested for weakness. The ulnar nerve should be palpated at the elbow to assess stability within the cubital tunnel, Tinel's, and potential sources of impingement.

Provocative maneuvers to assess the valgus stability include a static valgus stress test at 70° to 90°, the moving valgus stress test, and milk test. The moving valgus stress test has been the most accurate in predicting medial ulnar collateral ligament injury [12]. The elbow is brought through range of motion while the examiner applies a valgus force (Fig. 2). A positive correlative result is noted when the patient experiences pain at midrange of motion (70°–120°) when flexing and extending the elbow while applying valgus force [12]. The milk test is performed by having the patient reach with the contralateral hand under the affected elbow and grasp the ipsilateral thumb (Fig. 3). A valgus force is applied by the patient with the elbow flexed, and medial elbow pain with this maneuver indicates a positive result [13]. The lateral elbow also must be incorporated into the examination to ascertain radiocapitellar impaction or combined lateral instability. The ipsilateral shoulder of the throwing athlete must be examined for potential instability, impingement, rotator cuff strength, and scapular positioning, which could potentiate the medial elbow instability.

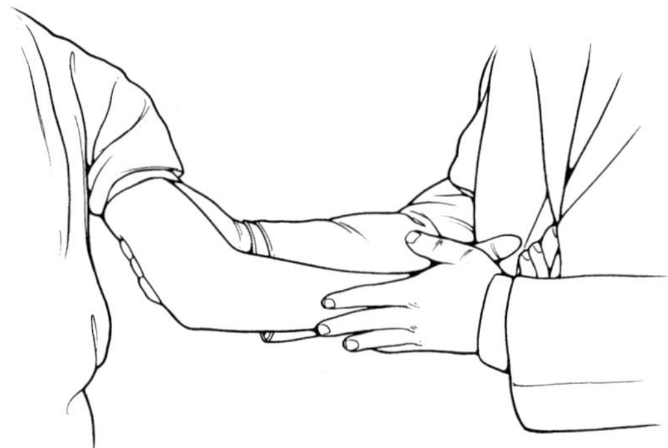

Fig. 2. "Moving valgus stress test" as described by O'Driscoll for valgus instability.

Orthop Clin N Am 39 (2008) 229–236

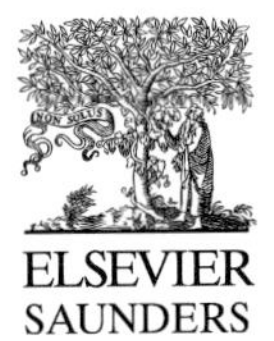

Olecranon Fractures

Christian J.H. Veillette, MD, MSc, FRCSC, Scott P. Steinmann, MD*

Department of Orthopedic Surgery, Mayo Clinic, 200 First Street, SW, Rochester, MN 55905, USA

Approximately 10% of fractures about the adult elbow consist of fractures of the olecranon process of the ulna and range from simple non-displaced fractures to complex fracture–dislocations of the elbow (Table 1). Several treatment options for internal fixation have been described, including tension-band wiring, plate fixation, intramedullary screw fixation, and triceps advancement after fragment excision. The method of internal fixation is chosen based primarily on fracture type. Because olecranon fractures are all intra-articular injuries, they require anatomic or essentially normal surface reduction and trochlear notch contour for predictable outcomes. In addition, fixation must be stable enough to permit early mobilization to avoid significant elbow stiffness. Given the variability in fracture patterns, the complex anatomy, and associated injuries, treating surgeons must be familiar with multiple treatment methods and follow a systematic surgical strategy to avoid complications and achieve reliable outcomes.

Anatomy

The elbow is a complex hinge joint that relies on a combination of bony articulations and soft tissue constraints to optimize stability and mobility [1]. Soft tissue constraints about the elbow are responsible for as much as 40% of the resistance to valgus stress and 50% of that to varus stress in the extended position. The anterior band of the ulnar collateral ligament acts as the major stabilizer to valgus stress. The major stabilizer to

varus or rotatory stress is the lateral collateral ligament complex, including the lateral ulnar collateral ligament [2,3].

The ulnohumeral articulation is the essential factor for osseous stability and mobility in the flexion–extension plane. The olecranon and coronoid processes comprise the semilunar or greater sigmoid notch of the ulna, which articulates with the trochlea. The olecranon blocks the anterior translation of the ulna with respect to the distal humerus, whereas an intact coronoid process resists posterior subluxation of the proximal ulna in extension beyond 30° or greater [4].

A transverse bare area devoid of cartilage is found at the midpoint between the coronoid and the tip of the olecranon [5]. This region must not be overcompressed during fracture reduction in an attempt to obtain articular cartilage reduction because this will result in a narrowed trochlear fossa and incongruent radius of curvature. The ossification center of the olecranon generally appears by 9 to 10 years of age, and fuses to the proximal ulna by 14 years of age. Persistence of the physis into adulthood may occur and can be confused with a fracture; clues to this condition include its familial tendency and common presence bilaterally. The triceps tendon inserts into the posterior third of the olecranon and is intimately associated with the periosteum. In addition, the triceps is continuous with the aponeurosis of the anconeus muscle and common extensor origin. Patella cubiti, an accessory ossicle embedded in the distal triceps, may be present and can be mistaken for a fracture [6].

The ulnar nerve passes around the posterior aspect of the medial epicondyle and between the two heads of the flexor carpi ulnaris, which spans in an arcade-like manner from the medial epicondyle to the olecranon process to form the

---

* Corresponding author.

E-mail address: steinmann.scott@mayo.edu (S.P. Steinmann).

0030-5898/08/$ - see front matter © 2008 Elsevier Inc. All rights reserved.
doi:10.1016/j.ocl.2008.01.002

orthopedic.theclinics.com

Table 1
Summary of olecranon fracture treatment based on displacement, comminution and joint stability

Classification	Description	Treatment
Mayo type IA and IB	Undisplaced (<2 mm) fractures with no comminution (IA) or with comminution (IIB)	Sling immobilization, early active range of motion, close follow-up
Mayo type IIA	Stable fractures with >3 mm displacement, no comminution	Tension band wiring usually adequate; consider plate and screw constructs if fracture lines are distal to coronoid; consider excision in low-demand patients or when small fragments are present
Mayo type IIB	Stable fractures with >3 mm displacement; comminution is present	Plate and screw constructs preferred, especially in patients <60 years old. Consider excision in low-demand patients or those >60 years, who have fractures with extensive comminution, or when small fragments are present
Mayo type IIIA	Unstable, displaced fracture–dislocations; no comminution is present	Plate-and-screw constructs preferred
Mayo type IIIB	Unstable, displaced fracture–dislocations; comminution is present	Plate and screw constructs preferred
Avulsion fractures		Tension band wiring or excision may be used

roof of the cubital tunnel. The nerve lies posterior to the ulnar collateral ligament, which forms the floor of the cubital tunnel and attaches in a fanlike fashion to the medial border of the olecranon. The brachialis tendon inserts broadly onto the proximal ulnar metaphysic distal to the tip of the midportion of the anterior coronoid.

Mechanism of injury

Fractures of the olecranon occur from either direct or indirect trauma. A fall or blunt trauma on the posterior tip of the elbow may cause fracture directly. Indirect avulsion of the olecranon from forces generated within the triceps muscle may occur with eccentric contraction during a fall on a partially flexed elbow. Amis and Miller [7] investigated the effect of impact mechanisms on olecranon fracture patterns in a cadaveric model. Radial head and coronoid fractures occurred from impact to the forearm with the elbow in 80° of flexion or less; olecranon fractures followed direct blows at 90° of flexion; and distal humerus fractures were caused by impact when the elbow was in greater than 110° of flexion. In cases of severe force to the elbow, a fracture dislocation can occur with posterior displacement of the olecranon fragment and the distal ulnar fragment together with the head of the radius anterior to the humerus.

Classification

The Mayo classification of olecranon fractures is based on three variables: displacement, stability, and comminution [8]. Type I fractures are nondisplaced, type II fractures are displaced but the ulnohumeral joint is stable, and type III fractures are displaced and unstable. Each fracture type is subdivided into noncomminuted (A) and comminuted fractures (B). Colton's [9] classification reflects displacement and the anatomy of the fracture, thus providing guidance as to the most biomechanically appropriate type of fixation. Fractures are described as nondisplaced and stable if they are displaced less than 2 mm and exhibit no change in position with gentle flexion to 90° or with extension against gravity. Displaced fractures can be further divided into avulsions fractures, transverse or oblique fractures, isolated comminuted fractures, or fractures with associated dislocations.

Diagnosis

History

Patients who have an olecranon fractures and associated injuries present with pain and swelling about the distal arm and elbow. Those who have displaced fractures have an obvious deformity, and attempted motion may elicit painful bony crepitus. The mechanism of injury and any associated neurovascular complications associated with the initial injury should be elicited from the patient. Thorough assessment for concurrent illnesses precipitating the injury and a detailed account of comorbid conditions is important.

Clinical examination

Physical examination should begin with assessment of the condition of the soft-tissues around the elbow. Extensive swelling, ecchymosis, and any abrasions or lacerations should be noted and may influence the timing of surgery. An assessment of range of motion or strength of the elbow should not be vigorously pursued. A palpable sulcus may be present at the site of an olecranon fracture, accompanied by a painful and limited range of motion. An important sign associated with isolated olecranon fractures is inability to extend the elbow actively against gravity. Although the pain associated with this maneuver may make patients hesitant to cooperate, this inability indicates discontinuity of the triceps mechanism. A careful neurovascular examination is essential, especially before any planned manipulation of the elbow.

Radiographic and imaging assessment

Plain radiographs in the anteroposterior, true lateral, and oblique projections are usually provide sufficient information for an accurate diagnosis. Severe comminution with displacement and overlap of the fracture fragments can obscure thorough determination of the fracture pattern. Thus, radiographs must be good quality, out of splint, and obtained while maintaining gentle longitudinal traction with inclusion of the elbow joint on the film. Poorly aligned radiographs performed in the splint are not as well suited for accurate diagnosis, classifying the fracture, and formal preoperative planning. Radiographs should be carefully evaluated for the presence of associated injuries, such as a radial head fracture or dislocation, a distal humerus fracture, or a coronoid fracture. Rarely does CT provide additional information that alters decision making, and preoperative planning with an isolated olecranon fracture and should be reserved for more complex fracture combinations.

Treatment

Nondisplaced fractures of the olecranon (Mayo type IA and IB) can be treated nonoperatively.

These fractures are defined by displacement less than 2 mm, no change in position with gentle flexion to 90°, or extension of the elbow against gravity. These fractures are immobilization in a long arm cast with the elbow in 90° of flexion for 3 to 4 weeks followed by protected range of motion exercises. Flexion past 90° should be avoided until bone healing is complete radiographically at approximately 6 to 8 weeks. In elderly patients, range of motion may be initiated earlier than 3 weeks if patients can tolerate it, with the goal to prevent stiffness. A follow-up radiograph should be obtained within 5 to 7 days after cast application to ensure that displacement of the fracture has not occurred. Immobilization in full extension is not recommended because stiffness is more likely, and fractures that require full extension for reduction should be treated operatively.

Tension band wire

Displaced olecranon fractures require operative treatment to restore elbow extension, joint congruity, and elbow stability. Transverse fractures without comminution (Mayo type IIA) are amenable to tension band wiring. The tension band wire construct converts the tensile distraction force of the triceps into a dynamic compressive force across the olecranon articular surface (Fig. 1). Traditionally, K-wires have been used in the tension band construct. Intramedullary cancellous screw fixation should be avoided in elderly patients who have underlying osteoporosis, because the proximal fragment may fracture further if a single 6.5-mm cancellous screw is used to secure the longitudinal component of the fracture.

Technique

Two 1.6-mm or 2.0-mm K-wires are inserted into the olecranon tip to obtain proximal control, and engagement distally in the anterior cortex of the ulna increases the stability of fixation [10]. Care should be taken to avoid overpenetration of the wires, because they may cause neurovascular damage, limitation in forearm rotation, or heterotopic ossification. The length of the wire should be noted at the point where it engages the second cortex. Once the wire penetrates the far cortex, it should be partially backed out and bent 180° at the previously noted position and cut. The fibers of the triceps tendon should be split sharply with a scalpel at the site of the K-wires to allow the cut and bent ends to be impacted against the cortex. A figure-of-8 loop of 1.5-mm or 18-gauge wire is positioned through a drill hole

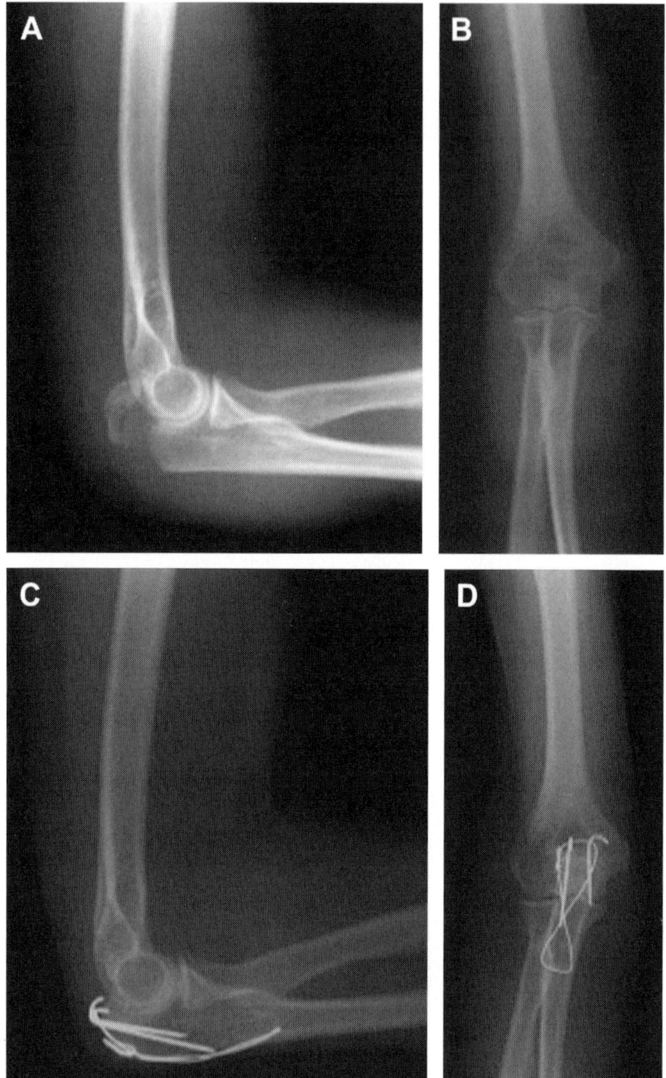

Fig. 1. This 60-year-old nurse practitioner fell while running and sustained a type IIA olecranon fracture (*A*, *B*). She underwent open reduction and internal fixation with tension band wiring (*C*, *D*). At latest follow-up she had range of motion from 10° to 100° in the flexion/extension arc. She complained of prominent hardware and underwent hardware removal at 20 months after her fracture fixation. (*From* Adams JE, Steinmann SP. Fractures of the Olecranon. In: Berry DJ, Steinmann SP. Adult reconstruction. Philadelphia: Wolters Kluwer Health/Lippincott Williams & Wilkins; 2007. p. 440; with permission.)

located distally approximately and equal distance from the fracture as the tip of the olecranon. The wire is then passed deep to the fibers of the triceps, adjacent to bone, beneath the K-wires. The wire is tightened by twisting in two places on opposite arms of the crossed portion of the figure-of-8 for additional stability. The K-wires are seated firmly in the bone using an impactor, beneath the fibers of the triceps to prevent wire migration.

In transverse fractures with comminution (Mayo type IIB), the tension band technique will collapse the fragments together, leading to a narrowed olecranon articulation that does not track properly. The most optimal fixation for these fractures is offered with contoured, limited-contract dynamic compression (LCDC) plate fixation, with or without bone graft depending on the size of the comminuted region [11]. Similarly, plate with lag screw fixation is preferred over the tension band construct for oblique fractures or unstable displaced olecranon fracture–dislocations with and without comminution (Mayo type IIIA and IIIB). Treatment with the tension band technique in this fracture pattern often results in displacement, because compression along the tension band causes shortening along the inclined plane of the obliquity or does not allow adequate fixation to restore stability and permit early mobilization.

Limited-contract dynamic compression plate fixation

Using the LCDC plate for fixation has several advantages [12,13]. The plate allows improved contouring and can be appropriately placed on the dorsal tension surface of the proximal ulna around the tip of the olecranon to help hold the proximal fragment when poor bone quality limits screw purchase (Fig. 2). The redesigned screw holes allow greater angulation of screw placement

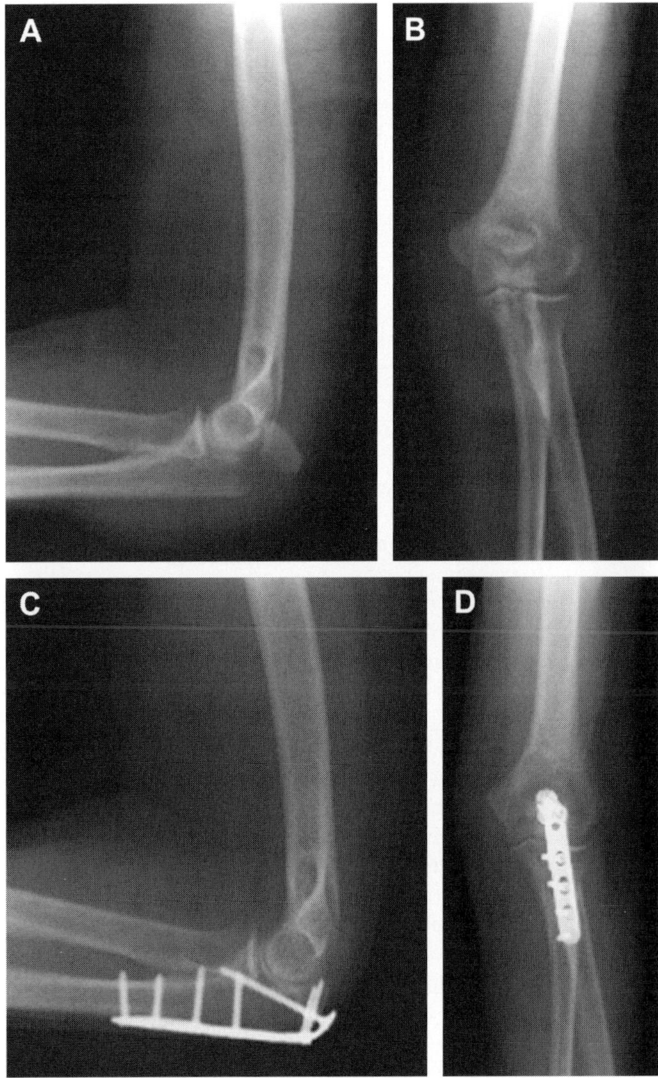

Fig. 2. This 66-year-old right-hand–dominant retired laboratory technician slipped on the ice and fell, sustaining a direct blow to her left elbow and this Mayo type IIA fracture of the olecranon (*A, B*). She underwent plate-and-screw osteosynthesis (*C, D*). At 18 months postoperatively, she was pain-free and her range of motion was 0° to 140°, with supination to 70° and pronation to 80°. (*From* Adams JE, Steinmann SP. Fractures of the Olecranon. In: Berry DJ, Steinmann SP. Adult reconstruction. Philadelphia: Wolters Kluwer Health/Lippincott Williams & Wilkins; 2007. p. 440; with permission.)

and the option of compression from either side of the screw hole. In addition, its lower profile allows its use in subcutaneous situations when soft tissue coverage may be in question. The proximal fixation of the plate is often the greatest challenge because the bone may be thin, and thus cancellous screws rather than cortical screws should be used in elderly patients. The advent of newer precontoured plates allows for an increased number of fixation points in the proximal fragment and cradles the olecranon along its dorsal surface. In complex fractures of the proximal ulna, a large coronoid fragment is often present. This fragment is very important to the final stability of the elbow and must be fixed with lag screws placed either through or adjacent to the implanted plate to prevent early posterior subluxation of the elbow [14]. Mobilizing the proximal olecranon fragment in the same way as an olecranon osteotomy allows the coronoid to be visualized and reduced through the olecranon fracture.

Technique

Patients are placed in a lateral position on the operating room table with the injured arm on a bolster across the chest. A sterile tourniquet is placed on the upper arm after skin preparation and draping. A posterior midline incision centered on the olecranon is extended proximally 5 cm from the tip of the olecranon. The ulna is approached along its subcutaneous border and the anconeus can be elevated to approach the radial head if required. Impacted articular fragments are elevated and the coronoid is then reduced and provisionally fixed to the ulna with one or two K-wires. The use of a heavy suture passed around the coronoid fragment can assist with temporary reduction. A narrow 3.5-mm LCDC plate is then contoured to fit the proximal ulna with the maximum bend, near 90°, between the second and third screw holes of the plate. The plate length must be able to accommodate three or four screws distal to the fracture. Once fracture reduction is achieved, the contoured plate is applied to the dorsal aspect of the olecranon and the triceps fascia is incised to allow the implant to sit on the bone. The plate is secured proximally with one screw from the fourth or fifth hole obliquely upward into the coronoid process. Fixation of the coronoid can also be performed or supplemented with lag screws adjacent to the plate. A long cancellous screw is placed from the first or second hole across the fracture toward the proximal shaft at the base of the coronoid.

Additional screws are placed proximally in the olecranon and the plate is secured distally to the shaft with three or four bicortical screws.

In the osteoporotic olecranon, direct trauma to the posterior aspect of the elbow can cause an isolated severely comminuted fracture. Excision of the fracture fragments and reattachment of the triceps tendon may be indicated in elderly patients whose olecranon fracture fragments are too small or too comminuted for successful internal fixation (Fig. 3). However, the coronoid and anterior soft tissues, collateral ligaments, and interosseus membrane must be intact, otherwise instability will result. The triceps tendon is reattached adjacent to the articular surface with nonabsorbable sutures that are passed through drill holes in the remaining proximal ulna. Reattaching the triceps this way creates a sling for the trochlea and a smooth congruent transition from the triceps tendon to the articular surface but decreases the moment arm, and may result in a weaker extensor mechanism but enhanced elbow stability [15]. The amount of olecranon that can be excised safely has been debated. Based on in vitro [4] and clinical studies [16,17] between 50% and 70% of the olecranon articular surface can be excised without compromising elbow stability provided the coronoid and distal trochlea are preserved.

Complications

Painful hardware irritation requiring removal is one of the most common complications after internal fixation of olecranon fractures. Complaints related to prominent hardware have been reported in up to 80% of cases. A higher incidence of prominent painful hardware has been reported after tension band wiring than compression plating [18,19]. Although Simpson and colleagues [12] reported no cases of symptomatic hardware irritation after LCDC plating, Bailey and colleagues [20] reported that 20% of patients required plate removal because of prominence of the plate fixation.

Loss of motion is rarely a significant problem in patients with isolated olecranon fractures. The typical lose of motion is 10° to 15° of extension in patients who have isolated injuries. However, patients who have associated fractures of the radial head or coronoid are more likely to develop limitations in their range of motion.

Nonunion of olecranon fractures have been reported in up to 1% of patients, with typical

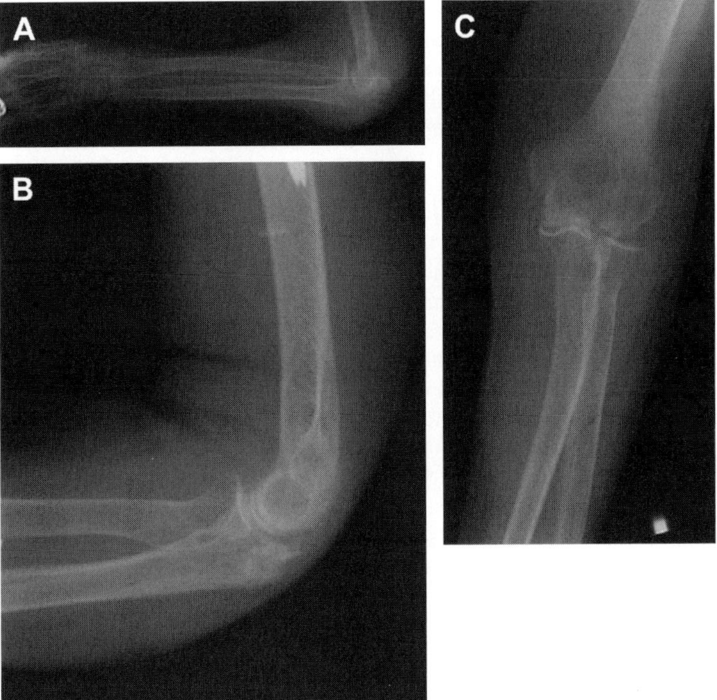

Fig. 3. This 84-year-old right-hand–dominant woman experienced a syncopal episode and fell down the stairs at home. She sustained concomitant fractures of the left proximal humerus, left distal radius, and left ulnar styloid, and a fracture of the left olecranon (*A*) treated with excision of the proximal fragment (*B, C*). At 6 months postoperatively, she was pain-free and her range of motion in the flexion extension arc was from 20° to 135°; pronation was to 70° and supination was to 70°. (*From* Adams JE, Steinmann SP. Fractures of the Olecranon. In: Berry DJ, Steinmann SP. Adult reconstruction. Philadelphia: Wolters Kluwer Health/Lippincott Williams & Wilkins; 2007. p. 440; with permission.)

symptoms of pain, instability, or loss of motion [21]. Treatment options for olecranon nonunions include excision, osteosynthesis with a LCDC plate, and bone graft or elbow arthroplasty in the presence of severe posttraumatic arthritis. Acceptable management of elderly patients includes excision of the proximal portion of the pseudarthrosis and repair of the triceps tendon, ensuring that the coronoid and anterior soft tissues are intact.

Rehabilitation

In elderly patients, early initiation of physical therapy is one of the most important issues in elbow surgery. An initial posterior plaster slab with the elbow flexed to 90° can be applied in the operating room to help manage immediate postoperative pain. The posterior slab is discontinued after 5 to 7 days and a removable splint is provided. Gentle active-assisted and passive motion is then started, with patients instructed to support the wrist with the opposite hand and gently flex and extend the elbow, gradually increasing the range of motion. Patients are instructed to take the arm out of the splint several times daily for these exercises and to let gravity work on extending the elbow. Active motion against resistance is avoided until callous formation is evident, usually at 8 to 10 weeks. If the stability of the fixation is a concern, then a hinged fracture brace can be used to provide additional support.

Results and outcome

Outcomes after olecranon fracture are generally good to excellent, with most series noting satisfactory outcomes and restoration of normal or near-normal function in more than 95% of patients.

Bailey and colleagues [20] evaluated the functional outcome of plate fixation for displaced olecranon fractures (Mayo type II or III) in 25 patients at an average of 34 months follow-up. Patient satisfaction was high (9.7/10) with a low pain rating (1/10). Based on the Mayo elbow score, 22 patients had excellent or good outcomes, and the mean DASH score showed almost normal upper extremity function.

Karlsson and colleagues [22] evaluated the long-term outcome of closed olecranon fractures in 73 patients at a mean of 19 years after fracture. Primary treatment consisted of open reduction and internal fixation in 84% of the elbows. Of these patients, 61 had no complaints at follow-up, 9 had occasional pain, and 3 had daily pain; 96% had an excellent or good overall outcome.

Summary

Olecranon fractures are commonly seen in orthopedic practice and have good to excellent outcomes with adherence to a treatment algorithm based on displacement, comminution, and joint stability. Although decreased range of motion, radiographic evidence of degenerative changes, and requirement for hardware removal are common, they can be minimized through careful attention to proper technique, anatomic reduction with stable fixation, and early mobilization.

References

[1] Morrey BF, An KN. Articular and ligamentous contributions to the stability of the elbow joint. Am J Sports Med 1983;11(5):315–9.

[2] O'Driscoll SW, Bell DF, Morrey BF. Posterolateral rotatory instability of the elbow. J Bone Joint Surg Am 1991;73(3):440–6.

[3] Cohen MS, Hastings H II. Rotatory instability of the elbow. The anatomy and role of the lateral stabilizers. J Bone Joint Surg Am 1997;79(2):225–33.

[4] An KN, Morrey BF, Chao EY. The effect of partial removal of proximal ulna on elbow constraint. Clin Orthop Relat Res 1986;209:270–9.

[5] Stormont TJ, An KN, Morrey BF, et al. Elbow joint contact study: comparison of techniques. J Biomech 1985;18(5):329–36.

[6] Winter M, Balaguer T, Tabutin J. Bilateral patella cubiti. A case report. J Bone Joint Surg Am 2006; 88(2):415–7.

[7] Amis AA, Miller JH. The mechanisms of elbow fractures: an investigation using impact tests in vitro. Injury 1995;26(3):163–8.

[8] Morrey BF. Current concepts in the treatment of fractures of the radial head, the olecranon, and the coronoid. Instr Course Lect 1995;44:175–85.

[9] Colton CL. Fractures of the olecranon in adults: classification and management. Injury 1973;5(2): 121–9.

[10] Prayson MJ, Williams JL, Marshall MP, et al. Biomechanical comparison of fixation methods in transverse olecranon fractures: a cadaveric study. J Orthop Trauma 1997;11(8):565–72.

[11] Hak DJ, Golladay GJ. Olecranon fractures: treatment options. J Am Acad Orthop Surg 2000;8(4): 266–75.

[12] Simpson NS, Goodman LA, Jupiter JB. Contoured LCDC plating of the proximal ulna. Injury 1996; 27(6):411–7.

[13] McKee MD, Seiler JG, Jupiter JB. The application of the limited contact dynamic compression plate in the upper extremity: an analysis of 114 consecutive cases. Injury 1995;26(10):661–6.

[14] Doornberg J, Ring D, Jupiter JB. Effective treatment of fracture-dislocations of the olecranon requires a stable trochlear notch. Clin Orthop Relat Res 2004;429:292–300.

[15] Coonrad RW, Morrey BF. Management of olecranon fractures and nonunion. In: Morrey BF, editor. Master techniques in orthopaedic surgery: the elbow. 2nd edition. Philadelphia: Lippincott Williams & Wilkins; 2002. p. 103–26.

[16] Inhofe PD, Howard TC. The treatment of olecranon fractures by excision or fragments and repair of the extensor mechanism: historical review and report of 12 fractures. Orthopedics 1993;16(12): 1313–7.

[17] Gartsman GM, Sculco TP, Otis JC. Operative treatment of olecranon fractures. Excision or open reduction with internal fixation. J Bone Joint Surg Am 1981;63(5):718–21.

[18] Hume MC, Wiss DA. Olecranon fractures. A clinical and radiographic comparison of tension band wiring and plate fixation. Clin Orthop Relat Res 1992;285:229–35.

[19] Wolfgang G, Burke F, Bush D, et al. Surgical treatment of displaced olecranon fractures by tension band wiring technique. Clin Orthop Relat Res 1987;224:192–204.

[20] Bailey CS, MacDermid J, Patterson SD, et al. Outcome of plate fixation of olecranon fractures. J Orthop Trauma 2001;15(8):542–8.

[21] Papagelopoulos PJ, Morrey BF. Treatment of nonunion of olecranon fractures. J Bone Joint Surg Br 1994;76(4):627–35.

[22] Karlsson MK, Hasserius R, Karlsson C, et al. Fractures of the olecranon: a 15- to 25-year followup of 73 patients. Clin Orthop Relat Res 2002;403:205–12.

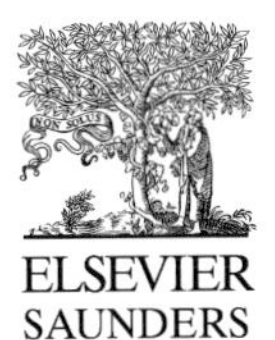

ELSEVIER
SAUNDERS

Orthop Clin N Am 39 (2008) 237–249

ORTHOPEDIC
CLINICS
OF NORTH AMERICA

Distal Biceps Rupture

Augustus D. Mazzocca, MD*, Jeffrey T. Spang, MD,
Robert A. Arciero, MD

*Department of Orthopaedic Surgery, University of Connecticut, John Dempsey Hospital,
Medical Arts and Research Building, 263 Farmington Avenue, Farmington, CT 06034-4037, USA*

The treatment of distal biceps ruptures has recently received increased scrutiny in the orthopedic community. The increasing demands of the middle-aged population and multiple advances in fixation methods have focused attention on improving outcomes and restoring function faster in patients treated operatively. In addition, newer treatment methods have the potential to decrease some of the complications noted with more traditional surgical techniques. Many of these newer techniques use single anterior incisions and apply hardware originally used in other areas of the body. Although nonoperative management is still beneficial in some patients, usually a successful repair of a ruptured distal biceps tendon can be combined with an aggressive early range-of-motion protocol to maximize function while minimizing time lost to injury.

Demographics

Rupture of the distal insertion of the biceps tendon remains an uncommon injury based on reported clinical series. Prior published papers have reported that only approximately 3% of biceps injuries involve the distal insertion [1,2]. More recent literature noted an incidence of 1.2 per 100,000 patients [3]. This same review by Safran and Graham [3] noted that the dominant extremity was most often involved (86% in the series) and the average age of the patient was 47 years. Other reviews of the literature have cited an average age of 50 years (range, 18–72 years) [4]. Safran's review

also noted a significantly higher rate of distal biceps rupture in smokers. Series [5–8] have reported a majority of male patients, but reports exist of female patients who had complete distal biceps injuries [8–10]. Rupture of the distal biceps has also been linked to anabolic steroid use [11] and bodybuilding [2].

Etiology

The pathophysiology preceding distal biceps rupture remains unclear. Although some patients report pain in the anterior elbow before an acute rupture, many experience no symptoms before the traumatic event. Early authors suggested that a bony prominence may lead to damage at the tendon insertion [12], but this may represent either a normal anatomic variant (Fig. 1) [13] or a bone spur secondary to another pathologic process. Morrey [14] hypothesized that irregularity of the radial tuberosity or bursitis may contribute to tendon degeneration before rupture. Other authors have speculated that mechanical impingement or the presence of a watershed (low arterial flow) area of the tendon may lead to tendon rupture [15]. Microscopic studies of tendons that ruptured, including the biceps tendon, have shown intrinsic degenerative changes [4], whereas some authors report degenerative changes in nearly all distal biceps tendon ruptures [16]. Some combination of anatomic factors and local tendon degeneration probably contribute to failure of the distal biceps tendon, although this has not been proven conclusively. The mechanism of injury is most often a single traumatic event characterized by an unexpected extension load applied to an elbow flexed to 90° [4]. Tears at the musculotendinous junction of the

---

* Corresponding author.

E-mail address: admazzocca@yahoo.com
(A.D. Mazzocca).

0030-5898/08/$ - see front matter © 2008 Elsevier Inc. All rights reserved.
doi:10.1016/j.ocl.2008.01.001

orthopedic.theclinics.com

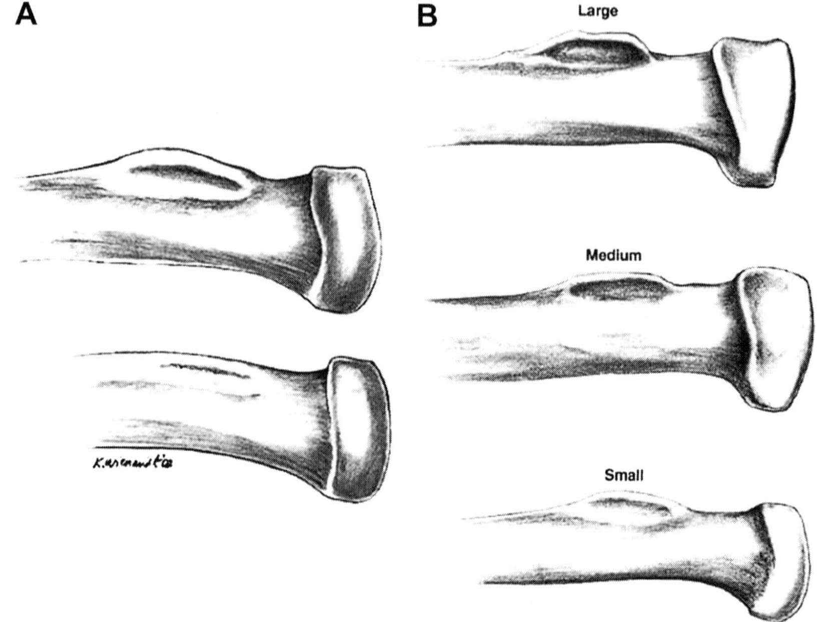

Fig. 1. (*A*) The bifid ridge type (*top*) has two prominent ridges, one medial and lateral, with a trough in between, whereas the smooth type has no ridge (*bottom*). (*B*) The single-ridge type was separated into three subtypes based on qualitative appearance: small, medium, and large. (*From* Mazzocca AD, Cohen M, Berkson E, et al. The anatomy of the bicipital tuberosity and distal biceps tendon. J Shoulder Elbow Surg 2007;16(1):124; with permission.)

distal biceps have been reported [17], and multiple authors report partial tears of the tendon [18–21], but in most cases the tendon avulsion is complete.

Clinical evaluation

Most patients can recall a single traumatic event and report a sudden sharp tearing pain in the anterior elbow region followed by discomfort in the lower arm. Occasionally patients may report pain in the posterolateral elbow. The intense pain usually relents in a few hours. Immediate weakness in flexion is common, but may diminish as the acute pain subsides [4,14]. If patients continue to use the extremity for physically demanding activities, they may report aching in the arm and forearm with repeated elbow flexion and supination.

Immediate postinjury physical examination can document ecchymosis in the antecubital fossa and occasionally over the proximal ulnar aspect of the elbow [14,19]. Tenderness is often present over the bicipital tuberosity and the distal arm. A defect can usually be palpated compared with the uninjured arm. The appreciable defect may be minimized if the bicipital aponeurosis remains intact, but careful examination will show a distinct

side-to-side difference. If the tendon seems to be in continuity but is tender to palpation, a partial biceps rupture should be considered [18]. Grinding or crepitus with forearm rotation may also be noted with partial tendon rupture [22]. Active flexion of the elbow results in retraction of the distal biceps, accentuating the deformity in complete ruptures. A thorough physical examination usually shows weakness in supination, and weakness with elbow flexion may also be evident early postinjury.

For patients who have a history and physical examination compatible with complete tendon rupture, a limited radiographic evaluation may be considered. Plain radiographs may show changes in the radial tuberosity [12] but generally do not change the treatment plan. If the physical examination and history are not conclusive, MRI should be considered. MRI may provide useful information about the integrity of the distal biceps tendon with respect to partial tendon ruptures, but may not change the treatment plan [20]. Other potential causes of pain in the antecubital fossa include cubital bursitis, bicipital tendonitis, partial biceps tendon rupture, and entrapment of the lateral antebrachial cutaneous nerve.

Classification

Classification of distal biceps tendon ruptures is descriptive and somewhat arbitrary. Ruptures may be defined as complete or partial based on tendon continuity. Acute ruptures have been defined as fewer than 4 weeks, with chronic ruptures defined as more than 4 weeks [4]. In reviewing chronic ruptures, ruptures may be further divided based on the presence of an intact bicipital aponeurosis or a ruptured aponeurosis. In theory, the intact aponeurosis may prevent extreme retraction of the tendon complex, making a later reinsertion of the injured tendon more feasible. For chronic ruptures without an intact aponeurosis, a soft-tissue grafting procedure may be required [23–25].

Treatment

Partial rupture

Partial rupture of the distal biceps tendon must be distinguished from the other causes of antecubital fossa pain to allow appropriate treatment. Most authors have reported case series of partial ruptures that were atraumatic [19,20,22], but a recent report showed most patients were able to recall a significant traumatic event [18]. In either case, nonoperative management may be attempted with a focus on stretching and strengthening. Symptoms may persist and some patients may experience functional limitations in elbow flexion and supination. Patients who do not experience response to nonoperative management may be considered for operative intervention. Although occasional cases have reported success with limited debridement [22], authors have reported consistent success with releasing the remaining tendon from the radial tuberosity and completing the procedure with a tendon reinsertion [14,18,20,21]. In one study, the authors used a posterior approach to successfully detach and repair the tendon, eliminating the need for an anterior exposure [26].

Complete rupture

Most patients will experience functional improvements if a complete rupture of the distal biceps tendon is repaired back to the radial tuberosity [4,14,27,28]. Studies have shown that patients treated operatively may experience return of full flexion and supination strength, whereas those treated nonoperatively do not experience complete return of function, particularly with repetitive activities [29]. Although the biceps is not the main elbow flexor, its contribution to

supination has been well documented [30]. One study comparing tenodesis of a ruptured distal biceps to the brachialis with anatomic repair noted excellent return of elbow flexion strength in the tenodesis group but significant weakness in supination compared with anatomic repair [31]. Nonoperative management should be reserved for low-demand patients who do not require normal flexion or supination strength or endurance, or whose other health issues raise the risk of operative treatment to unacceptable levels.

Techniques

Historically, repair techniques used an extensile anterior incision to reinsert the avulsed tendon. This method led to unacceptably high rates of radial nerve injury [32] and prompted Boyd and Anderson [33] to develop a two-incision technique designed to minimize risk to the neurovascular structures in proximity to the radial tuberosity. This approach was successful in lowering the risk for serious nerve injury, but repairs were complicated by the presence of heterotopic ossification and radioulnar synostosis. Morrey and colleagues [27] modified the original Boyd-Anderson technique to avoid subperiosteal dissection using a muscle-splitting approach to try to decrease the rate of serious heterotopic ossification and synostosis. However, this modification did not eliminate the complications of heterotopic ossification or postoperative nerve paresthesias [34], and interest in alternative methods of fixation continued to develop. The advent of suture anchors renewed the interest in the single anterior incision approach to distal biceps tendon repairs, and current techniques may be broadly divided into two-incision or single anterior incision techniques.

Two-incision technique

Morrey's modification to the Boyd-Anderson technique has been well described (Fig. 2) [14,27]. A transverse 3- to 4-cm incision is made over the anterior aspect of the elbow, the deep fascia is incised, with care taken to identify and protect the lateral antebrachial cutaneous nerve, and the distal biceps tendon is located. If the bicipital aponeurosis remains intact, it will often tether the distal biceps and keep it from retracting. During this dissection multiple vessels are encountered and must be cauterized or ligated to clear the surgical approach to the radial tuberosity. The stump of the distal biceps must be located and a nonabsorbable suture is passed so that its ends emerge on the

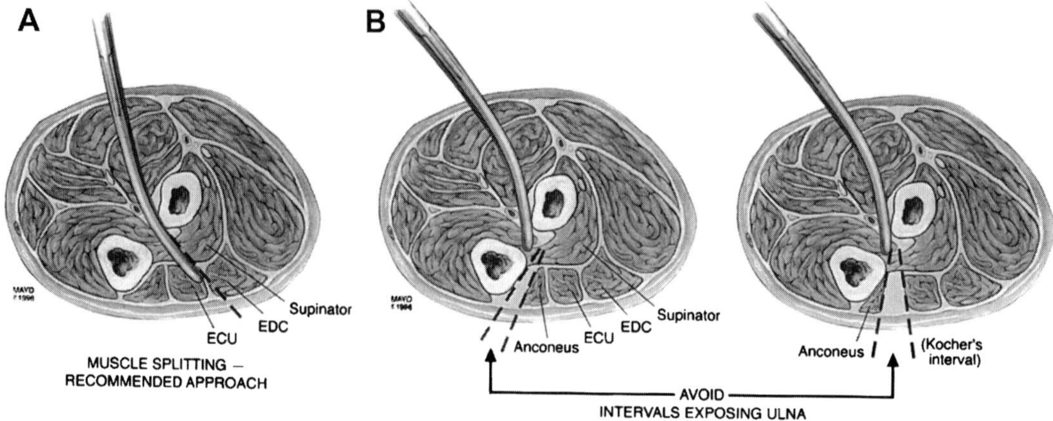

Fig. 2. (*A*) The curved hemostat passes close to the radius and past the tuberosity, avoiding the ulna. (*B*) Curving the instrument toward the ulna is to be avoided. ECU, extensor carpi ulnaris; EDC, extensor digitorum communis. (*From* Morrey BF. Injury of the flexors of the elbow: biceps tendon injury. In: Morrey BF, editor. The elbow and its disorders. 3rd edition. Philadelphia: Saunders; 2000. p. 474; with permission.)

avulsed surface. Multiple acceptable options for tendon-grasping sutures have been described, including Bunnell or Krackow configurations. If the rupture is treated acutely, the tendon sheath should be intact, making blunt dissection down to the radial tuberosity possible. At this point, the forearm is fully supinated and a blunt hemostat is advanced along the medial border of the radial tuberosity to the dorsolateral aspect of the proximal forearm [4]. It is vital to avoid violating the periosteum of the ulna. The elbow is flexed and a second posterior incision is made over the hemostat down to the fascia, covering the common extensor muscle mass. This muscle mass and the supinator muscle are split down to the radial tuberosity, with the forearm rotated into maximum pronation. Pronation of the forearm protects the deep branch of the radial nerve as it traverses the substance of the supinator and brings the radial head into view. A burr may be used to create

a trough in the radial tuberosity large enough to accept the distal biceps tendon, while two to three holes are drilled in the margin to accept sutures (Fig. 3A, B). The sutures in the distal biceps tendon are passed from anterior to posterior and the tendon is delivered deep and medial to the lateral antebrachial cutaneous nerve. Passage of the sutures through the drill holes draws the tendon into the trough and provides firm fixation.

Before hardware developments, which stimulated interest in single anterior approach techniques, the modified Boyd-Anderson approach was the standard approach used for distal biceps reconstruction. Excellent clinical results have been reported by multiple authors [2,6,14,29,35–37]. Of note, Cheung and colleagues [36] reported recently on a postoperative protocol using immediate range of motion, without deleterious effects on healing or strength. Although traditionally patients were immobilized in the immediate postoperative period [4], more

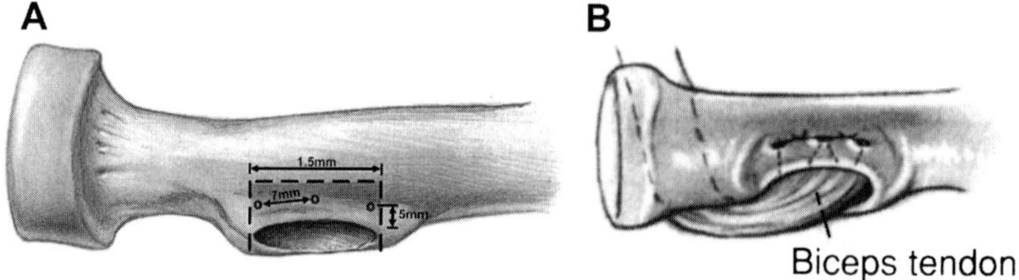

Fig. 3. (*A*) Osseous bridges 5 to 7 mm from the edge and 7 mm between the holes are ideal and the biceps tendon is then brought through its previous tract (*B*) and reinserted into the radial tuberosity with two nonabsorbable sutures. (*From* Morrey BF. Injury of the flexors of the elbow: biceps tendon injury. In: Morrey BF, editor. The elbow and its disorders. 3rd edition. Philadelphia: Saunders; 2000. p. 473; with permission.)

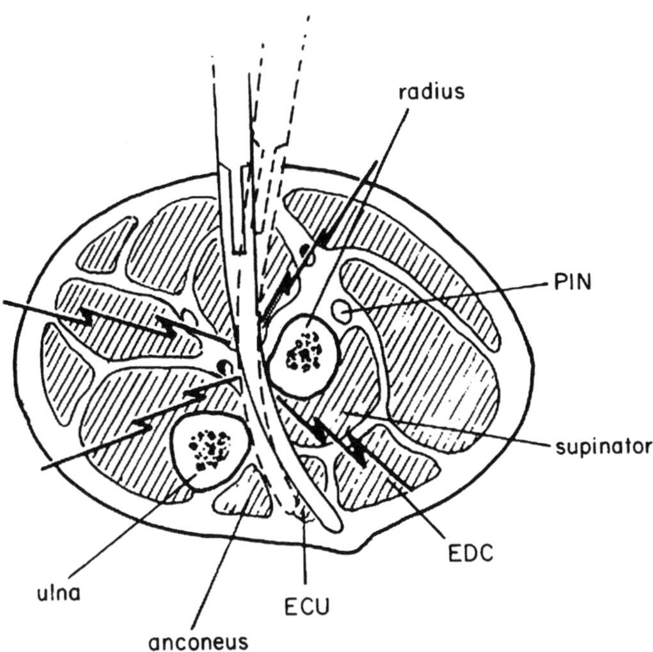

Fig. 4. Potential mechanism of synostosis formation with the two-incision technique for repair of distal biceps tendon rupture. The dotted outline of the instrument represents potential contact with bones and thereby creates a path along which synostosis may develop. ECU, extensor carpi ulnaris; DC extensor digitorum communis; PIN, posterior interosseous nerve. (*From* Sotereanos DG, Sarris I, Chou KH. Radioulnar synostosis after the two-incision biceps repair: a standardized treatment protocol. J Shoulder Elbow Surg 2004;13(4):449; with permission.)

aggressive range-of-motions protocols may be possible using a standard Morrey modification of the Boyd-Anderson technique.

Complications

Complications with the modified Boyd-Anderson technique have been reported in multiple clinical reports and case studies [5,27,38,39]. In general, reported complications may be broadly grouped into heterotopic ossification leading to radioulnar synostosis and nerve injuries. Although careful dissection and a muscle-splitting technique may minimize the risk for radioulnar synostosis (Fig. 4), this is a recognized complication of the

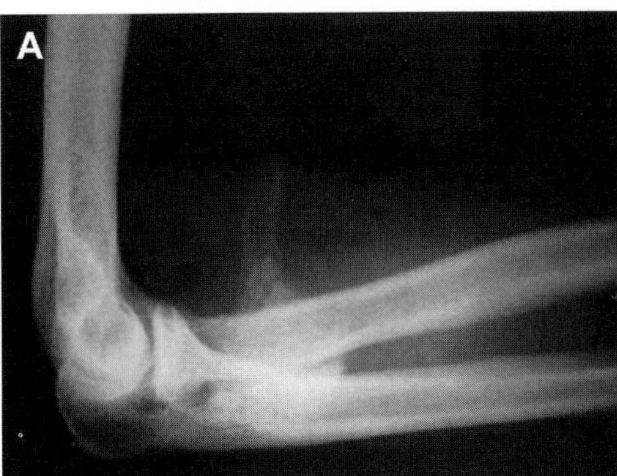

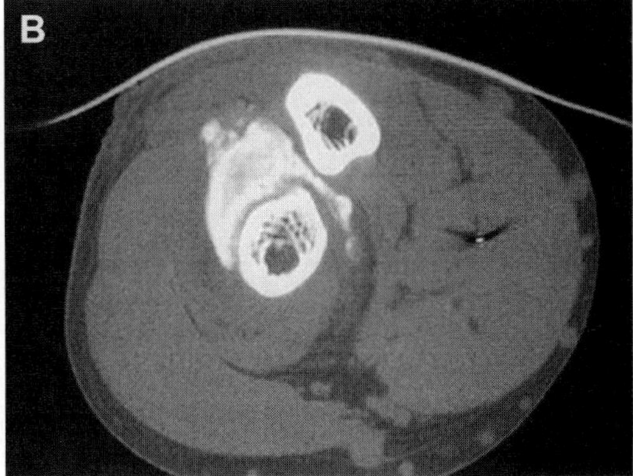

Fig. 5. Lateral radiograph (*A*) and CT scan (*B*) of radioulnar synostosis 9 months after distal biceps repair with the two-incision technique. (*From* Sotereanos DG, Sarris I, Chou KH. Radioulnar synostosis after the two-incision biceps repair: a standardized treatment protocol. J Shoulder Elbow Surg 2004;13(4):450; with permission.)

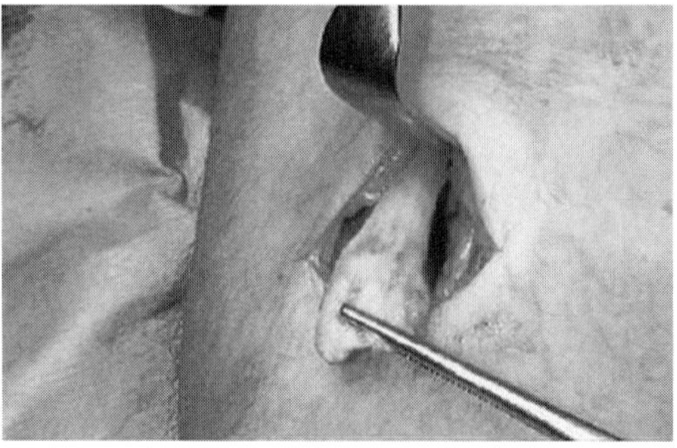

Fig. 6. A single anterior incision centered over the bicipital tuberosity is made, and subcutaneous dissection proximally allows the distal stump to be retrieved. (*From* McKee MD, Hirji R, Schemitsch EH, et al. Patient-oriented functional outcome after repair of distal biceps tendon ruptures using a single-incision technique. J Shoulder Elbow Surg 2005;14(3):303; with permission.)

Boyd-Anderson surgical approach (Fig. 5A, B) [34,40]. Because of the proximity of multiple neurovascular structures, care must be taken with any anterior elbow approach, and nerve injury is not a complication unique to the two-incision technique. Multiple case studies note injury to major nerves, including the lateral antebrachial cutaneous, posterior interosseous, and median nerve, with a two-incision technique [41–43].

Single anterior incision

To avoid the dissection associated with the standard two-incision format, techniques were developed to approach the radius through a single anterior incision. Early reports focused on the placement of suture anchors in the radial tuberosity for distal biceps tendon fixation [44–48]. Recent reports have described the use of an Endobutton (Smith and Nephew, Andover, Massachusetts) or interference screws in conjunction with a single anterior approach [49–51]. One report even describes a technique combining endoscopic viewing of the distal biceps tendon with Endobutton fixation [52].

The approach to the proximal radius is similar to the anterior portion of the two-incision technique but may need to be expanded to appropriately visualize the radial tuberosity for tendon reinsertion. As with the two-incision technique, the biceps tendon is delivered out of the wound for tendon preparation and eventual suturing (Fig. 6).

Suture anchor

The suture anchor technique relies on fixation at the radial tuberosity and a suturing construct that maximizes tendon apposition with the radial tuberosity (Fig. 7A, B). Some authors recommend creating a trough for tendon insertion [7], whereas others recommend only lightly abrading the anterior cortex before inserting the suture anchor (Fig. 8A, B) [8]. The authors of each study reported excellent results for more than 60 patients treated with suture anchor repairs. These findings mirror the earlier reports of excellent clinical outcomes using suture anchor techniques [44–46].

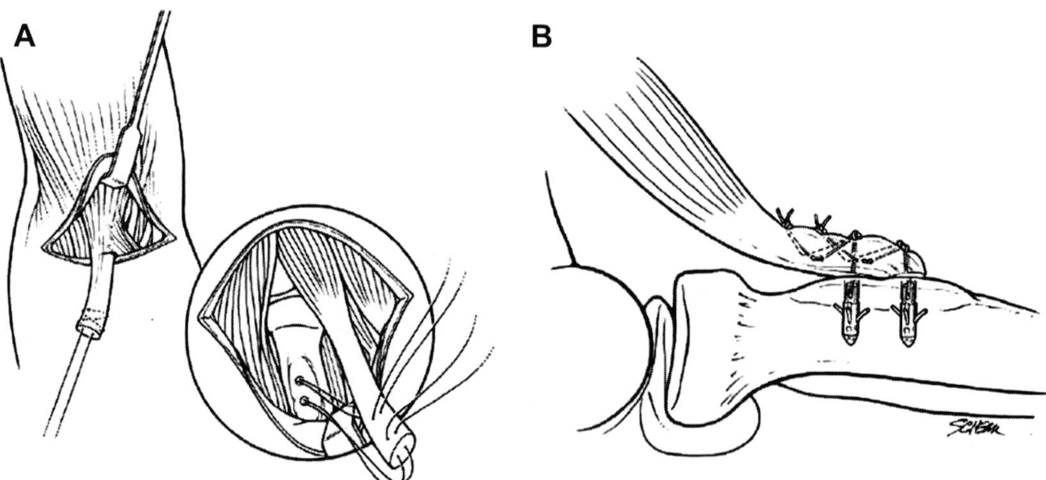

Fig. 7. Suture passage (*A*) and knot tying (*B*) used to achieve stable reapproximation of biceps tendon. (*From* John CK, Field LD, Weiss KS, et al. Single-incision repair of acute distal biceps ruptures by use of suture anchors. J Shoulder Elbow Surg 2007;16(1):80; with permission.)

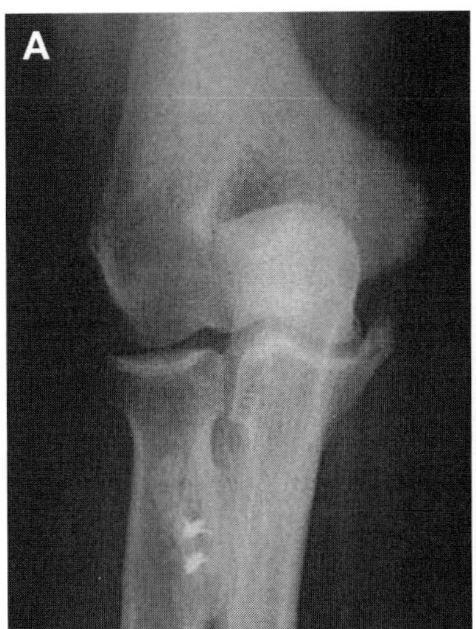
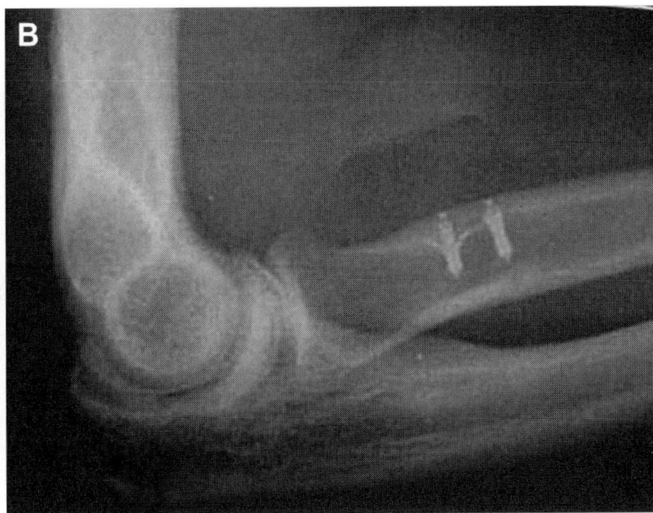

Fig. 8. Anteroposterior (*A*) and lateral (*B*) radiographs showing suture anchor placement into radial tuberosity. (*From* John CK, Field LD, Weiss KS, et al. Single-incision repair of acute distal biceps ruptures by use of suture anchors. J Shoulder Elbow Surg 2007;16(1):80; with permission.)

Benefits of suture anchor fixation include the easy availability of suture anchors in the surgical setting and surgeon familiarity with suture anchors for soft-tissue fixation.

Endobutton

Bain and colleagues [49] initially described a repair method using an Endobutton and a bony trough to reattach the distal biceps tendon. Subsequently, Greenberg and colleagues [50] reported on some limited mechanical studies and included a clinical report that showed excellent early results. This technique uses a standard anterior approach and creates a trough in the radial tuberosity to accept the tendon. The tendon is attached to the Endobutton outside the surgical wound (Fig. 9) and then passed through a small hole drilled in the posterior cortex of the radius. The Endobutton is then flipped to draw the tendon into the bone trough (Fig. 10A–C). Fixation is achieved by engaging the posterior cortex of the radius (Fig. 11). Limited clinical results have been reported.

Interference screw

Mazzocca and colleagues [51,53] reported on two techniques using a biointerference screw. One technique suggests using only a biointerference screw and the other combines screw fixation with the Endobutton technique previously

described. For each technique the tendon is connected to the cannulated screwdriver–screw construct by threading one suture attached to the distal biceps tendon through the interference screw. The tendon is then guided into the trough

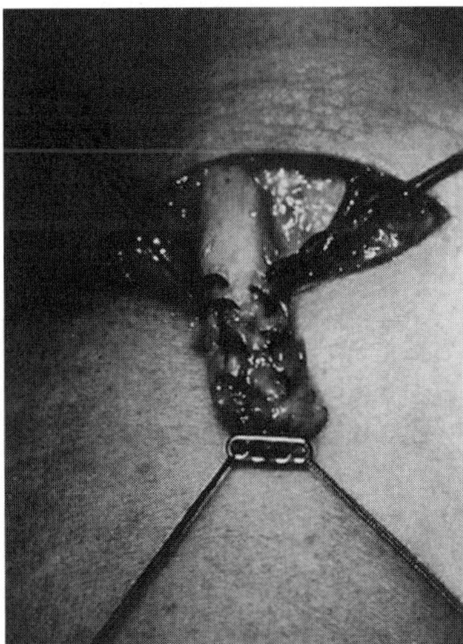

Fig. 9. Biceps tendon is delivered through incision, and two Bunnell 5/0 Ethibond sutures fix Endobutton. With leading and trailing sutures attached, tendon is "prefabricated." (*From* Bain GI, Prem H, Heptinstall RJ, et al. Repair of distal biceps tendon rupture: a new technique using the Endobutton. J Shoulder Elbow Surg 2000;9(2):121; with permission.)

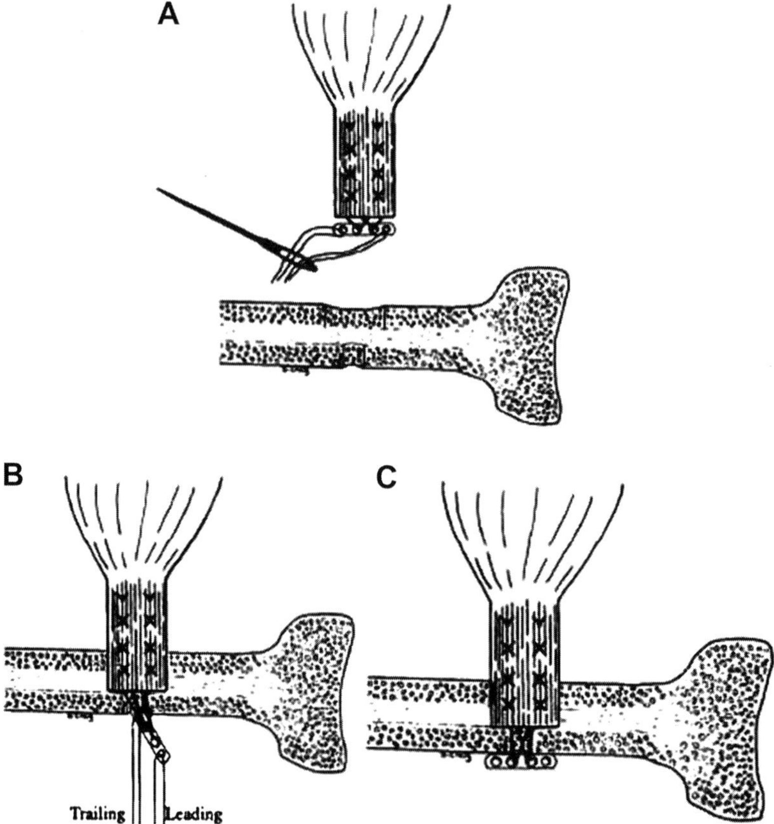

Fig. 10. (*A*) Straight-eyed needle with leading and trailing sutures. (*B*) Endobutton advances tendon into intramedullary canal of radius under fluoroscopic control. (*C*) Endobutton locks tendon into position and leading and trialing sutures are removed. (*From* Bain GI, Prem H, Heptinstall RJ, et al. Repair of distal biceps tendon rupture: a new technique using the Endobutton. J Shoulder Elbow Surg 2000;9(2):121; with permission.)

and the interference screw is placed on the ulnar side of the tendon, pushing the repaired tendon toward the radial side. Once the screw is inserted, the suture passing through the screw is tied back to a second suture in the distal biceps tendon (Fig. 12A, B). No clinical trials have been reported using interference screw techniques.

Complications

Most complications reported in the largest clinical series from single anterior approach techniques involve nerve injury to either the posterior interosseous nerve (PIN) or the lateral antebrachial cutaneous nerve (LAC) [7,8]. These nerves may be injured by overaggressive or prolonged retraction (PIN or LAC) or direct trauma during the surgical approach (LAC). Heterotopic ossification has been reported with the suture

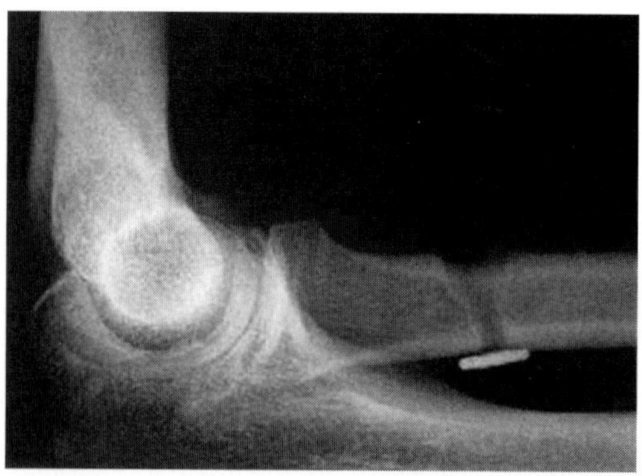

Fig. 11. Lateral radiograph showing the EndoButton locked and engaged on the posterior radial cortex. Note the preparation of the anterior radius. (*From* Greenberg JA, Fernandez JJ, Wang T, et al. EndoButton-assisted repair of distal biceps tendon ruptures. J Shoulder Elbow Surg 2003;12(5):486; with permission.)

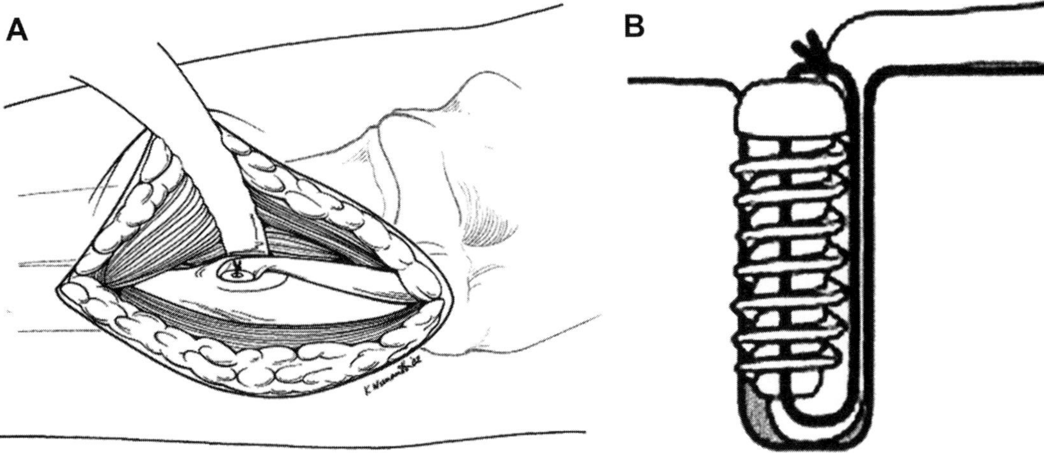

Fig. 12. The completed tenodesis with the distal biceps tendon on the ulnar aspect of the tuberosity possessing interference and suture anchor fixation. (*From* Mazzocca AD, Alberta FG. Single incision technique using an interference screw for the repair of distal biceps tendon ruptures. Oper Tech Sports Med 2003;11(1):40; with permission.)

anchor (Fig. 13) and Endobutton techniques (Fig. 14) [8,54]. Most authors have recommended aggressive irrigation after radial cortex preparation to try to limit heterotopic ossification.

Biomechanical studies

Increasing interest in alternatives to the modified Boyd-Anderson two-incision technique for distal biceps tendon repair led to multiple biomechanical comparisons. This substantial amount

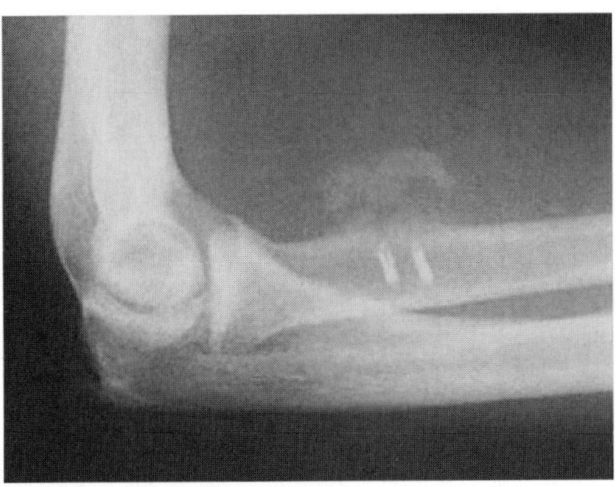

Fig. 13. Radiograph showing ectopic bone formation adjacent to distal biceps repair site. (*From* John CK, Field LD, Weiss KS, et al. Single-incision repair of acute distal biceps ruptures by use of suture anchors. J Shoulder Elbow Surg 2007;16(1):81; with permission.)

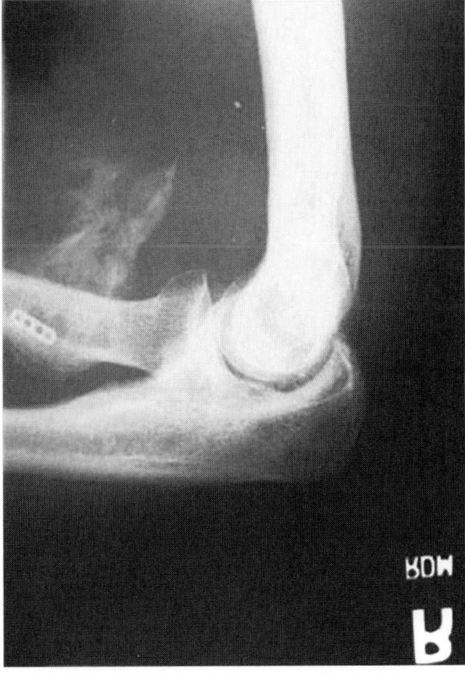

Fig. 14. Heterotopic ossification of the biceps tendon on lateral radiograph (*From* Agrawal V, Stinson MJ. Case report: heterotopic ossification after repair of distal biceps tendon rupture utilizing a single-incision EndoButton technique. J Shoulder Elbow Surg 2005;14(1):107; with permission.)

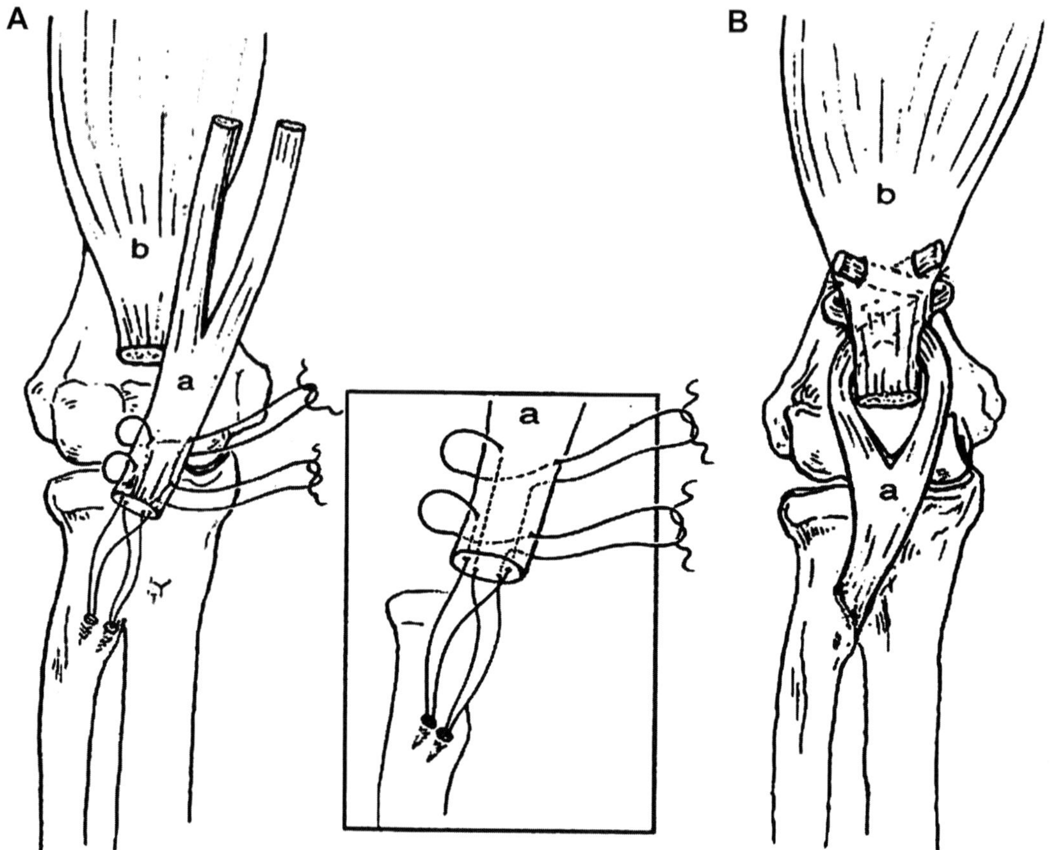

Fig. 15. (A) Schematic of the modified Kessler sliding stitch used to secure the Achilles tendon allograft (a) to the bicipital tuberosity. (B) Schematic of the Pulvertaft weave used to secure the Achilles tendon allograft (a) to the distal biceps stump (b). (*From* Darlis NA, Sotereanos DG. Distal biceps tendon reconstruction in chronic ruptures. J Shoulder Elbow Surg 2006;15(5):617; with permission.)

of biomechanical research has evolved as technical options have increased for tendon fixation. Early studies comparing bone tunnel (bone bridge) fixation and suture anchor fixation noted significant weaknesses in strength and stiffness for suture anchor constructs [55,56]. These findings did not dampen enthusiasm for the suture anchor technique, because failure loads were still believed to be sufficient to achieve stable healing of the tendon. A later study with more modern anchors concluded that suture anchor fixation may actually exceed the strength of bone tunnel fixation [57]. Greenberg and colleagues [50] compared bone tunnels, suture anchors, and Endobutton fixation in a nonanatomic model and found Endobutton to be significantly stronger. These investigators also measured the force required to pull an intact forearm from elbow extension to

flexion against gravity and found the largest specimen required 123 N for this range of motion. Although this finding does not consider muscle forces generated from active firing, it provides an estimate of the force a repair may encounter in the immediate postoperative period with simple range of motion.

A more recent anatomic model of tendon repair noted no statistically significant differences between the strength of Endobutton fixation and suture anchor fixation [58]. To evaluate intact tendon and repair techniques, Idler and colleagues [59] compared intact specimens with repair groups using bone tunnels or interference screws. They concluded that interference screw fixation more closely approximated the biomechanical profile of the intact distal biceps tendon. Krushinski and colleagues [60] compared interference screw versus suture anchor repairs and also concluded that the interference screw model was stronger and stiffer.

In the most comprehensive test to date, Mazzocca and colleagues [61] compared four different methods of distal biceps repair biomechanically (bone tunnel, Endobutton, suture anchor, and interference screw), and the Endobutton had a significantly greater load to failure than any other repair method. Failure loads ranged from 232 N (suture anchor) to 440 N (Endobutton).

Chronic rupture

Most authors consider early anatomic repair to be standard treatment for distal biceps tendon ruptures. Surgical treatment may be delayed because of error in diagnosis or a trial of nonoperative management. If treatment is delayed greater then 4 weeks after the initial injury, surgical repair is complicated. Patients may experience persistent pain and weakness, particularly with supination.

Mobilization of the retracted tendon may allow anatomic reinsertion into the radial tuberosity or the distal tendon may be inserted into the brachialis, but this nonanatomic repair has clear drawbacks [31]. Late biceps repair using an interposing graft has been proposed as a more anatomic alternative (Fig. 15A, B) [62]. For each surgical procedure, an extensile incision is required to release the distal biceps and achieve access to the radial tuberosity. Multiple graft sources have been cited in the literature for the interposition, including flexor carpi radialis [63], Achilles tendon allograft [23,62], autograft semitendinosis [24,64], and semitendinosis with Endobutton fixation [65]. Small clinical reports have accompanied the description of each technique and satisfactory results have been reported, making late reconstruction of the distal biceps with an interposition graft a viable option.

Summary

Rupture of the distal biceps tendon can lead to pain and limitations with elbow flexion and supination. Historically, nonoperative management or nonanatomic repairs reportedly yielded acceptable results, but anatomic reinsertion has become standard treatment for most patients in the acute setting. Multiple techniques have yielded excellent clinical outcomes, including the traditional two-incision technique and the single anterior incision technique. With the recent advances in hardware, alternative fixation methods with single anterior incision approaches are being explored. Biomechanical studies of these newer methods are encouraging, but limited clinical reports are available. More aggressive rehabilitation regimens for all surgical techniques have led to increased patient satisfaction and maximized results. Even in chronic cases, anatomic repairs of the distal biceps tendon have led to encouraging clinical results. Increasing patient follow-up has shown that orthopedic surgeons have multiple reasonable options for distal biceps repair.

References

[1] Gilcreest E, Albi P. Unusual lesions of muscles and tendons of the shoulder girdle and upper arm. Surg Gynecol Obstet 1939;68(1939):903–17.

[2] D'Alessandro DF, Shields CL Jr, Tibone JE, et al. Repair of distal biceps tendon ruptures in athletes. Am J Sports Med 1993;21(1):114–9.

[3] Safran MR, Graham SM. Distal biceps tendon ruptures: incidence, demographics, and the effect of smoking. Clin Orthop Relat Res 2002;404:275–83.

[4] Ramsey ML. Distal biceps tendon injuries: diagnosis and management. J Am Acad Orthop Surg 1999; 7(3):199–207.

[5] Dobbie R. Avulsion of the lower biceps brachii tendon: analysis of fifty-one previously unreported cases. Am J Surg 1941;51:662–83.

[6] Karunakar MA, Cha P, Stern PJ. Distal biceps ruptures. A followup of Boyd and Anderson repair. Clin Orthop Relat Res 1999;363:100–7.

[7] McKee MD, Hirji R, Schemitsch EH, et al. Patient-oriented functional outcome after repair of distal biceps tendon ruptures using a single-incision technique. J Shoulder Elbow Surg 2005;14(3):302–6.

[8] John CK, Field LD, Weiss KS, et al. Single-incision repair of acute distal biceps ruptures by use of suture anchors. J Shoulder Elbow Surg 2007;16(1):78–83.

[9] Toczylowski HM, Balint CR, Steiner ME, et al. Complete rupture of the distal biceps brachii tendon in female patients: a report of 2 cases. J Shoulder Elbow Surg 2002;11(5):516–8.

[10] Bauman JT, Sotereanos DG, Weiser RW. Complete rupture of the distal biceps tendon in a woman: case report. J Hand Surg [Am] 2006;31(5):798–800.

[11] Visuri T, Lindholm H. Bilateral distal biceps tendon avulsions with use of anabolic steroids. Med Sci Sports Exerc 1994;26(8):941–4.

[12] Davis WM, Yassine Z. An etiological factor in tear of the distal tendon of the biceps brachii: report of two cases. J Bone Joint Surg Am 1956;38(6):1365–8.

[13] Mazzocca AD, Cohen M, Berkson E, et al. The anatomy of the bicipital tuberosity and distal biceps tendon. J Shoulder Elbow Surg 2007;16(1):122–7.

[14] Morrey BF. Injury of the flexors of the elbow: biceps in tendon injury. In: Morrey BF, editor. The elbow and its disorders. 3rd edition. Philadelphia: W.B. Saunders; 2000. p. 468–78.

[15] Seiler JG III, Parker LM, Chamberland PD, et al. The distal biceps tendon. Two potential mechanisms involved in its rupture: arterial supply and mechanical impingement. J Shoulder Elbow Surg 1995; 4(3):149–56.

[16] Postacchini F, Puddu G. Subcutaneous rupture of the distal biceps brachii tendon; a report on seven cases. J Sports Med Phys Fitness 1975;15(2):81–90.

[17] Schamblin ML, Safran MR. Injury of the distal biceps at the musculotendinous junction. J Shoulder Elbow Surg 2007;16(2):208–12.

[18] Dellaero DT, Mallon WJ. Surgical treatment of partial biceps tendon ruptures at the elbow. J Shoulder Elbow Surg 2006;15(2):215–7.

[19] Nielsen K. Partial rupture of the distal biceps brachii tendon. A case report. Acta Orthop Scand 1987; 58(3):287–8.

[20] Rokito AS, McLaughlin JA, Gallagher MA, et al. Partial rupture of the distal biceps tendon. J Shoulder Elbow Surg 1996;5(1):73–5.

[21] Vardakas DG, Musgrave DS, Varitimidis SE, et al. Partial rupture of the distal biceps tendon. J Shoulder Elbow Surg 2001;10(4):377–9.

[22] Bourne MH, Morrey BF. Partial rupture of the distal biceps tendon. Clin Orthop Relat Res 1991; 271:143–8.

[23] Darlis NA, Sotereanos DG. Distal biceps tendon reconstruction in chronic ruptures. J Shoulder Elbow Surg 2006;15(5):614–9.

[24] Hang DW, Bach BR Jr, Bojchuk J. Repair of chronic distal biceps brachii tendon rupture using free autogenous semitendinosus tendon. Clin Orthop Relat Res 1996;(323):188–91.

[25] Kaplan FT, Rokito AS, Birdzell MG, et al. Reconstruction of chronic distal biceps tendon rupture with use of fascia lata combined with a ligament augmentation device: a report of 3 cases. J Shoulder Elbow Surg 2002;11(6):633–6.

[26] Kelly EW, Steinmann S, O'Driscoll SW. Surgical treatment of partial distal biceps tendon ruptures through a single posterior incision. J Shoulder Elbow Surg 2003;12(5):456–61.

[27] Morrey BF, Askew LJ, An KN, et al. Rupture of the distal tendon of the biceps brachii. A biomechanical study. J Bone Joint Surg Am 1985;67(3):418–21.

[28] Agins HJ, Chess JL, Hoekstra DV, et al. Rupture of the distal insertion of the biceps brachii tendon. Clin Orthop Relat Res 1988;234:34–8.

[29] Baker BE, Bierwagen D. Rupture of the distal tendon of the biceps brachii. Operative versus nonoperative treatment. J Bone Joint Surg Am 1985; 67(3):414–7.

[30] Gordon KD, Pardo RD, Johnson JA, et al. Electromyographic activity and strength during maximum isometric pronation and supination efforts in healthy adults. J Orthop Res 2004;22(1):208–13.

[31] Klonz A, Loitz D, Wohler P, et al. Rupture of the distal biceps brachii tendon: isokinetic power analysis and complications after anatomic reinsertion compared with fixation to the brachialis muscle. J Shoulder Elbow Surg 2003;12(6):607–11.

[32] Meherin J, Kilgore E. The treatment of ruptures of the distal biceps brachii tendon. Am J Surg 1960; 99:636–40.

[33] Boyd H, Anderson L. A method for reinsertion of the distal biceps brachii tendon. J Bone Joint Surg Am 1961;43:1041–3.

[34] Kelly EW, Morrey BF, O'Driscoll SW. Complications of repair of the distal biceps tendon with the modified two-incision technique. J Bone Joint Surg Am 2000;82(11):1575–81.

[35] Davison BL, Engber WD, Tigert LJ. Long term evaluation of repaired distal biceps brachii tendon ruptures. Clin Orthop Relat Res 1996;333: 186–91.

[36] Cheung EV, Lazarus M, Taranta M. Immediate range of motion after distal biceps tendon repair. J Shoulder Elbow Surg 2005;14(5):516–8.

[37] Hovelius L, Josefsson G. Rupture of the distal biceps tendon. Report of five cases. Acta Orthop Scand 1977;48(3):280–2.

[38] Leighton MM, Bush-Joseph CA, Bach BR Jr. Distal biceps brachii repair. Results in dominant and nondominant extremities. Clin Orthop Relat Res 1995; 317:114–21.

[39] Failla JM, Amadio PC, Morrey BF, et al. Proximal radioulnar synostosis after repair of distal biceps brachii rupture by the two-incision technique. Report of four cases. Clin Orthop Relat Res 1990; 253:133–6.

[40] Sotereanos DG, Sarris I, Chou KH. Radioulnar synostosis after the two-incision biceps repair: a standardized treatment protocol. J Shoulder Elbow Surg 2004;13(4):448–53.

[41] Stearns KL, Sarris I, Sotereanos DG. Permanent posterior interosseous nerve palsy following a two-incision distal biceps tendon repair. Orthopedics 2004;27(8):867–8.

[42] Lin KH, Leslie BM. Surgical repair of distal biceps tendon rupture complicated by median nerve entrapment. A case report. J Bone Joint Surg Am 2001; 83(5):741–3.

[43] Katzman BM, Caligiuri DA, Klein DM, et al. Delayed onset of posterior interosseous nerve palsy after distal biceps tendon repair. J Shoulder Elbow Surg 1997;6(4):393–5.

[44] Lintner S, Fischer T. Repair of the distal biceps tendon using suture anchors and an anterior approach. Clin Orthop Relat Res 1996;322:116–9.

[45] Sotereanos DG, Pierce TD, Varitimidis SE. A simplified method for repair of distal biceps tendon ruptures. J Shoulder Elbow Surg 2000;9(3):227–33.

[46] Lynch SA, Beard DM, Renstrom PA. Repair of distal biceps tendon rupture with suture anchors. Knee Surg Sports Traumatol Arthrosc 1999;7(2):125–31.

[47] El-Hawary R, Macdermid JC, Faber KJ, et al. Distal biceps tendon repair: comparison of surgical techniques. J Hand Surg [Am] 2003;28(3):496–502.

[48] Morrison KD, Hunt TR III. Comparing and contrasting methods for tenodesis of the ruptured distal biceps tendon. Hand Clin 2002;18(1):169–78.

[49] Bain GI, Prem H, Heptinstall RJ, et al. Repair of distal biceps tendon rupture: a new technique using the Endobutton. J Shoulder Elbow Surg 2000;9(2):120–6.

[50] Greenberg JA, Fernandez JJ, Wang T, et al. Endo-Button-assisted repair of distal biceps tendon ruptures. J Shoulder Elbow Surg 2003;12(5):484–90.

[51] Mazzocca AD, Romeo AA, Alberta FG, et al. Single incision technique using an interference screw for the repair of distal biceps tendon ruptures. Oper Tech Sports Med 2003;11(1):36–41.

[52] Sharma S, MacKay G. Endoscopic repair of distal biceps tendon using an EndoButton. Arthroscopy 2005;21(7):897, e1–e4.

[53] Mazzocca AD, Bicos J, Arciero RA, et al. Repair of distal biceps tendon ruptures using a combined anatomic interference screw and a cortical button. Techniques in Shoulder and Elbow Surgery 2005;6(2):108–15.

[54] Agrawal V, Stinson MJ. Case report: heterotopic ossification after repair of distal biceps tendon rupture utilizing a single-incision Endobutton technique. J Shoulder Elbow Surg 2005;14(1):107–9.

[55] Berlet GC, Johnson JA, Milne AD, et al. Distal biceps brachii tendon repair. An in vitro biomechanical study of tendon reattachment. Am J Sports Med 1998;26(3):428–32.

[56] Pereira DS, Kvitne RS, Liang M, et al. Surgical repair of distal biceps tendon ruptures: a biomechanical comparison of two techniques. Am J Sports Med 2002;30(3):432–6.

[57] Lemos SE, Ebramzedeh E, Kvitne RS. A new technique: in vitro suture anchor fixation has superior yield strength to bone tunnel fixation for distal biceps tendon repair. Am J Sports Med 2004;32(2):406–10.

[58] Spang JT, Weinhold PS, Karas SG. A biomechanical comparison of EndoButton versus suture anchor repair of distal biceps tendon injuries. J Shoulder Elbow Surg 2006;15(4):509–14.

[59] Idler CS, Montgomery WH III, Lindsey DP, et al. Distal biceps tendon repair: a biomechanical comparison of intact tendon and 2 repair techniques. Am J Sports Med 2006;34(6):968–74.

[60] Krushinski EM, Brown JA, Murthi AM. Distal biceps tendon rupture: Biomechanical analysis of repair strength of the Bio-Tenodesis screw versus suture anchors. J Shoulder Elbow Surg Nov 8, 2007;16(2):218–23.

[61] Mazzocca AD, Burton KJ, Romeo AA, et al. Biomechanical evaluation of 4 techniques of distal biceps brachii tendon repair. Am J Sports Med 2007;35(2):252–8.

[62] Sanchez-Sotelo J, Morrey BF, Adams RA, et al. Reconstruction of chronic ruptures of the distal biceps tendon with use of an Achilles tendon allograft. J Bone Joint Surg Am 2002;84(6):999–1005.

[63] Levy HJ, Mashoof AA, Morgan D. Repair of chronic ruptures of the distal biceps tendon using flexor carpi radialis tendon graft. Am J Sports Med 2000;28(4):538–40.

[64] Wiley WB, Noble JS, Dulaney TD, et al. Late reconstruction of chronic distal biceps tendon ruptures with a semitendinosus autograft technique. J Shoulder Elbow Surg 2006;15(4):440–4.

[65] Hallam P, Bain GI. Repair of chronic distal biceps tendon ruptures using autologous hamstring graft and the Endobutton. J Shoulder Elbow Surg 2004;13(6):648–51.

ORTHOPEDIC
CLINICS
OF NORTH AMERICA

Orthop Clin N Am 39 (2008) 251–264

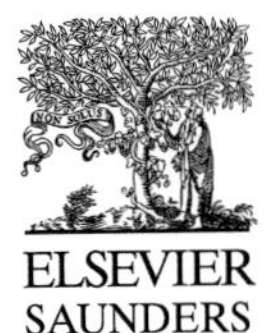

Soft Tissue Coverage of the Elbow: A Reconstructive Algorithm

Mark Jensen, MD[a], Steven L. Moran, MD[b,c],*

[a]Department of General Surgery, Mayo Clinic, 200 First Street SW, Rochester, MN 55905, USA
[b]Division of Plastic Surgery, Mayo Clinic, 200 First Street SW, Rochester, MN 55905, USA
[c]Department of Orthopedic Surgery, Mayo Clinic, 200 First Street SW, Rochester, MN 55905, USA

Soft tissue defects surrounding the elbow require reconstruction with thin, pliable, and durable tissue, which can withstand and allow for repetitive flexion and extension. In addition, optimal functional recovery in traumatic elbow injuries requires early, and in many cases, immediate motion to prevent stiffness and contracture. Historically, soft tissue coverage around the elbow has used local and distant donor tissue [1,2]. Coverage choices may include primary closure, skin grafting, local cutaneous flaps, fasciocutaneous transposition flaps, island fascial or fasciocutaneous flaps, muscle or myocutaneous pedicled flaps, and microvascular free-tissue transfer [1–3]. Despite the multitude of options for coverage, the authors have found four flaps to provide reliable coverage for most elbow deficits within their practice; these flaps are the latissimus dorsi flap, the radial forearm flap, the anconeus flap, and the anterior lateral thigh flap. This article provides an overview of treatment options for elbow coverage with emphasis on the use of these four specific flaps.

General principles

The ultimate choice of flap coverage depends on several variables, including size and complexity of the wound, exposure of vital structures, comorbid status of the patient, potential donor site morbidity, and overall outcome potential of the joint. Historically, the reconstructive algorithm for providing elbow coverage has proceeded in a step ladder fashion, with the simplest procedures being used first, before more complicated options (Box 1); however, with advancements in microsurgical techniques, the surgical procedure is often chosen over the reconstructive ladder, because it provides the patient with the best form and function.

In general, most elbow wounds that require coverage are located posteriorly. Defects located anteriorly, over the antecubital area, may often be covered with local fasciocutaneous flaps or simple skin grafts without significant compromise to motion. Coverage of posterior defects requires flaps that are thin and pliable and will allow for immediate motion. Hence, distant pedicled flaps (such as the thoracoepigastric flap) that require the elbow to be tethered to the chest wall should be discouraged because these promote edema and stiffness, in addition to requiring multiple procedures to provide definitive closure of the defect. If possible, the flap should provide sensate coverage to protect the elbow from long-term repetitive trauma and pressure-induced ulceration.

Patient assessment and timing of coverage

Soft tissue defects of the elbow should not be considered in isolation. Numerous patient factors affect the treatment plan and may limit reconstructive options. Traumatic defects are frequently associated with life-threatening injuries that need to be managed before wound reconstruction. Shock, acute lung injury, and ongoing organ failure will dictate a conservative approach. In contrast, aggressive reconstruction can be pursued in cases of isolated elbow injuries.

* Corresponding author.
E-mail address: moran.steven@mayo.edu
(S.L. Moran).

orthopedic.theclinics.com

Box 1. Reconstructive ladder

Primary closure
Secondary intention healing
Split-thickness skin graft
Full-thickness skin graft
Random pattern local flap
Axial pattern local flap
Island pattern local flap
Distant random pattern flap
Distant axial pattern flap
Free-tissue transfer [10]

In many cases, traumatic wound coverage can be performed in the first 24 hours after an initial thorough debridement. Early wound coverage, within the first 24 to 72 hours, is associated with decreased edema, lower wound infection rates, and less wound contraction, scar formation, pain, and limb dysfunction [2,4]. High-energy injuries, such as crush wounds, electric burns, avulsions, and grossly contaminated wounds, may require serial debridement to allow assessment of tissue viability. These wounds may be treated with open packing, temporary biologic dressings, or wound vacuum-assisted closure (VAC) therapy (V.A.C., KCI, San Antonio, Texas) until the wound is free of devitalized tissue, at which point the wound may be closed [5,6].

Systemic diseases frequently impact the choice of reconstruction because some disease processes can increase the risk of flap failure. Immunosuppression, chemotherapy, steroid use, radiation, collagen-vascular disorders, and smoking impede wound healing and can lead to an increased rate of wound complications. In particular, previous radiation exposure to the elbow may significantly compromise the viability of local pedicled flaps [7]. It has been the authors' preference in such cases to opt for free-tissue transfer because this method prevents any additional injury to the affected extremity and brings well-vascularized tissue to the site of injury. In elective cases of surgically created wounds, systemic illnesses and modifiable risk factors should be controlled in advance of surgery. Ideally, patients should quit smoking at least 1 month before surgical reconstruction [2,8–10].

Surgical planning

The major factors determining flap choice are location, size, and tissue involvement. Wounds with exposed muscle and subcutaneous tissue will accept skin grafts; however, exposure of vital structures such as tendon devoid of paratenon, nerve, vessels, bone, and hardware require flap coverage. Flap coverage is also indicated in situations where restoration of sensation or padding over a bony protuberance is needed, where a skin graft would be susceptible to breakdown. Composite flaps may be useful for the reconstruction of multiple component loss, such as bone and skin, or muscle and nerve [1,9–11].

Primary closure

Primary closure is indicated for small wounds where the skin can be approximated in a tension-free manner, with no underlying bone, joint, dead space, or hardware. Undermining the skin edges helps to bring the skin together, but care must be taken not to compromise capillary networks. Scar orientation should be considered to avoid subsequent joint contracture. Complications of primary closure include skin necrosis, infection, contracture, wound breakdown, and seroma [2,5,10,12].

Skin grafting

Skin grafting is indicated for wounds with an appropriate bed in locations not exposed to the risk of repetitive trauma. Acceptable beds for grafting include subcutaneous tissue, muscle, and paratenon. Wound beds that are grossly contaminated or infected or contain devitalized tissue will not support grafts. Skin grafts should not be used where repeated surgical procedures are suspected, such as bone grafting or nerve grafting. Special consideration is given to the location of skin grafts with respect to joint movement because scar contractures can lead to decreased elbow function.

Compared with full-thickness skin grafts, split-thickness grafts can cover large surface areas more easily and have a lower rate of primary graft loss, but will undergo a greater degree of secondary contracture over time [2,10,13–16]. Skin grafts are secured to the wound bed with chromic sutures or staples and covered by a nonadherent occlusive dressing. Grafts may be secured to the wound bed with the use of a tie-over cotton bolster. Alternatively, a wound VAC can be placed at 75 mm Hg constant suction for 5 days. If the VAC is used to secure the graft elbow, motion can begin on postsurgical day 1. If a standard bolster is used for graft immobilization, the graft is allowed to mature for 5 to 7 days before unrestricted motion of the elbow [13,16,17].

Skin grafts may work in conjunction with primary closure to cover small- to moderate-sized defects; if undermining of the surrounding tissue allows for a portion of the elbow wound to be closed primarily, skin grafting can be performed at the distal or proximal margins of the wound over the triceps or extensor muscle bellies (Fig. 1). Skin grafting will not work well if it lies directly over the olecranon. The major downside of skin grafting around the posterior surface of the elbow is secondary contracture, which may limit motion, in addition to the immobilization time necessary for graft take. Other short-term complications of skin grafting include donor site infections, graft loss, and scarring at the donor site [15–17].

Flap options

Flap terminology

Classification schemes for surgical flaps may be based on perfusion pattern, vascular anatomy, tissue components used, and donor site location. Flaps are characterized as axial or random, based on perfusion patterns. Axial flaps are perfused by a named central blood vessel, whereas random pattern flaps rely on an unnamed vascular plexus. Flaps may have their base proximal or distal to the wound bed. Proximally based flaps are referred to as antegrade flaps, whereas distally based

flaps are termed retrograde flaps. Axial flaps are sometimes named after the supplying artery or location of donor site; the radial forearm flap is an example. Composite flaps incorporate multiple tissue types, including bone, fascia, muscle, nerve, and skin. Vascular free flaps are divided and reanastomosed to local vasculature. Regardless of the classification scheme used, a sound understanding of vascular patterns should guide flap design. Failures generally relate to ischemia due to poor planning, or a lack of understanding of the vascular flow patterns [1–3,18,19].

Local random flaps

Local random flaps are indicated for small defects where the adjacent skin is healthy and viable. These flaps carry their own blood supply through dermal and subdermal plexuses and occasionally through a specific cutaneous artery. They should be designed in a 1:1 length-to-width ratio to avoid necrosis. Care must be taken in tissue handling to avoid injury to the capillary networks. Numerous flap designs are described, including advancement flaps, rotational flaps, Z-plasties, and rhomboid flaps. Secondary defects often require skin grafting. Rhomboid flaps are occasionally useful about the elbow when the defect is small and can be excised into a triangular shape. A rhombus with 60° and 120° angles is optimal but other angles may be accommodated. Tension at the flap tip and the donor site closure line presents limitations to this design. Double-Z rhomboid flap design

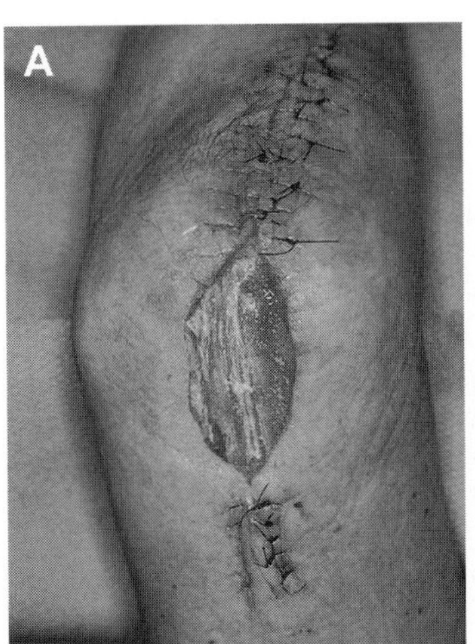
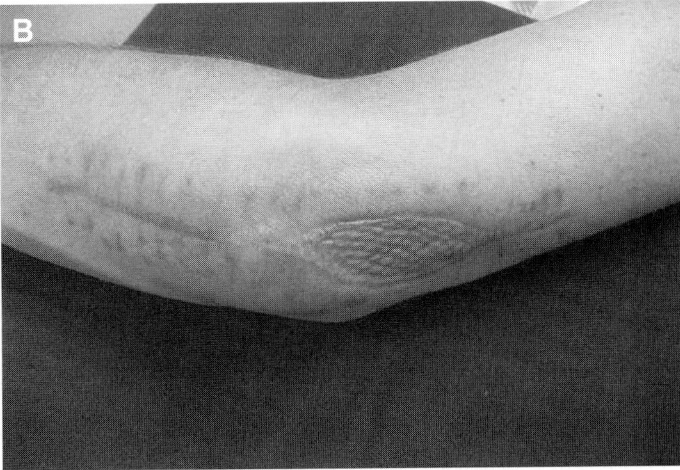

Fig. 1. (*A*) A posterior cutaneous defect overlying the triceps insertion, olecranon, and proximal ulna. (*B*) Undermining and local skin advancement allowed the wound to be closed over most of the olecranon and proximal ulnar; the remaining area could then be skin grafted with a split-thickness graft.

may be a superior alternative. Overall, these flaps are limited in their mobility and in their ability to cover large defects because of a poor random blood supply. When in doubt, it is better to use vascularized flaps rather than burn bridges with a failed local random flap [2,9,10,19,20].

Axial fasciocutaneous flaps

In contrast to random local flaps, axial fasciocutaneous flaps have the advantage of inclusion of a known axial blood supply, which allows for further extension in mobility and narrowing of the flap base to improve coverage. Blood supply to the skin of the upper extremity is served by a predictable pattern of cutaneous angiosomes, which can be used in planning local flaps. Blood vessels enter the skin from direct cutaneous vessels, musculocutaneous perforators, or fasciocutaneous vessels. These form subdermal and deep fascial plexuses. Inclusion of both plexuses improves flap survival. Axial flaps to the elbow are based on four dominant arteries. The brachial artery divides in the antecubital fossae to form the radial and ulnar arteries. The ulnar artery quickly gives off the common interosseous artery, which further divides into the posterior and anterior interosseous arteries. Together, the radial, ulnar, anterior, and posterior interosseous arteries give off fasciocutaneous perforators to supply the skin of the forearm at regular intervals. These form the basis for retrograde flaps to the elbow. It is important to ensure patent vascular arcades in the wrist and palm to allow retrograde flow through the ulnar and radial arteries when sacrificing one of these arteries for a flap. Antegrade flaps to the elbow are based on the rich collaterals about the elbow. In the lateral arm, the deep brachial artery anastomoses with the radial recurrent artery and recurrent interosseous artery. The inferior and superior ulnar collateral arteries anastomose with the anterior and posterior ulnar recurrent arteries, respectively [2,21–26].

The most common axial fasciocutaneous flap for elbow coverage is the radial forearm flap. Other options for pedicled axial fasciocutaneous coverage of the elbow include the retrograde lateral arm flap [23,27–30], the antecubital fasciocutaneous flap [2,25,31,32], the ulnar forearm flap, and the posterior interosseous flap.

Radial forearm island flap

The radial forearm flap has been the workhorse flap for elbow coverage because of its large size, reliability, and versatility. It is an orthograde flap, based on the radial artery. Nine to 17 perforating vessels supply the skin overlying the radial two thirds and lateral aspect of the anterior forearm. It has a large arc of rotation that extends the entire length of the radial artery to its origin 10 cm below the elbow joint; occasionally, the radial artery may have a proximal take-off from the brachial artery above the antecubital fossa. Flaps as large as 15 × 25 cm can be raised, but generally, flaps smaller than 8 × 16 cm are used for elbow coverage. It can be raised as a composite flap to include a portion of the distal radius, proximal brachioradialis muscle, flexor carpi radialis (FCR) muscle, or palmaris longus tendon. Sensibility to the flap is provided by the medial and lateral antebrachial cutaneous nerves. A complete palmar arch is mandatory to maintain perfusion to the hand through the ulnar and sometimes the median arteries following radial artery harvest. A patent superficial arch is verified with an Allen's test before flap elevation. If the radial forearm flap must be used in a patient without a patent arch, the radial artery can be reconstructed with the use of a saphenous vein graft. Reports of thumb ischemia have been reported in cases of incomplete palmar arches [26,33].

The main drawback to this flap is the high incidence of donor site morbidity and sacrifice of the radial artery. Richardson found in a series of 100 patients that 13% developed exposed tendons, 19% had delayed donor site healing, and 32% had decreased sensation in the radial nerve distribution. Radial fractures have been noted following bone harvest. These morbidities can be reduced by elevating a pure facial flap, reducing tendon exposures by dissecting superficially, using tissue expansion to allow primary closure of donor site, or using ulnar-based flaps to cover the donor site [22,23,34–38]. Despite donor site complications, the radial forearm flap has remained a workhorse flap for elbow coverage.

Technique

After a timed Allen's test, the course of the radial artery is marked with the help of a handheld Doppler probe [2,10,25]. The donor skin is marked larger than the defect and as distal as needed to allow the flap to reach the elbow. If the flap can be designed more proximal in the wrist and forearm, the resultant defect is easier to cover with skin grafting because more muscle belly is available to cover the surrounding tendon. Flap dissection is performed with the use of an upper arm tourniquet.

Flap dissection begins medially and proceeds toward the FCR. Once the FCR is identified, dissection begins laterally. Here, care is taken to preserve the radial dorsal sensory nerve. The cephalic vein is included with the flap, in addition to the later antebrachial cutaneous nerve, to allow for additional venous outflow and preservation of some sensation within the flap. Once the brachioradialis is identified, the radial artery can be identified within the septum between the FCR and brachioradial tendons. The distal radial artery and venous comitant are then ligated and divided, and the flap is then raised distal to proximal, including the antebrachial fascia, radial vessels, and fasciocutaneous perforators. Care is taken to preserve paratenon over the FCR and brachioradialis for subsequent grafting. The flap is raised on its pedicle and transposed to cover the elbow defect. Donor site closure requires a skin graft. The authors prefer to use a nonmeshed graft to improve cosmesis. The wrist and digits are then immobilized with a splint for 5 to 7 days to prevent partial skin graft loss (Fig. 2).

Pedicle muscle flaps

The use of muscle flaps in elbow coverage is preferred when infection is present or when dead space to be filled is significant. Muscle flaps can provide more bulk than fasciocutaneous flaps, which can help to obliterate dead space. Historically, it has been thought that muscle provides for improved outcomes in cases of infection [39,40]. In addition to providing coverage, muscle flaps may be transferred to restore elbow flexion. Elbow flexion may be restored with either a pedicled latissimus dorsi or triceps transfer. Other commonly used muscle flaps about the elbow include the brachioradialis, flexor carpi ulnaris, and anconeus [41,42]. The authors have found the anconeus and latissimus to be the most frequently used muscle flaps in their institution [43].

Anconeus flap

The anconeus is a small muscle in the posterolateral forearm that originates at the lateral epicondyle and inserts on the proximal ulna. The vascular anatomy and technique for transfer of this muscle were delineated by Mathes and Nahai [44] in 1982 and Parry and colleagues [25] 1988. This size and location of the muscle make it a useful option for coverage of small- to medium-sized defects over the radiocapitellar joint, the distal triceps tendon, and the olecranon [45]. Its blood supply is primarily through the recurrent posterior interosseus and medial collateral arteries [25,45]. Functionally, this muscle helps to provide the terminal 15° of elbow extension and supination of the forearm; its harvest results in little to no functional deficits. Transfer is facilitated by a blood supply that enters proximally, underneath the muscle, allowing expeditious transposition and rotation to posterior defects of the elbow.

The anconeus's usefulness is limited by its small size and short pedicle, which do not allow coverage of anterior or medial defects. In addition, the muscle's blood supply can be sacrificed inadvertently when exposing the elbow with the posterior-lateral approach for open reduction and internal fixation of comminuted fractures. Complications are few and the flap may be harvested under regional blockade in patients who would not tolerate a general anesthetic [25,45].

Technique

The fascia overlying the lateral proximal portion of the ulna is elevated to reveal the anconeus muscle. Dissection begins medially to separate the muscle from its ulnar attachments. The muscle may then be divided distally and the undersurface of the muscle can be visualized and the pedicle isolated. The medial collateral artery, a branch of the profunda brachii, enters proximally. Once the vascular pedicle is visualized, dissection continues over the lateral and proximal margins of the muscle. Islanding the muscle on its vascular pedicle alone can facilitate transfer more proximally and to the medial surface of the elbow (Fig. 3).

Latissimus dorsi myocutaneous pedicle flap

The latissimus dorsi muscle flap has been the workhorse flap for elbow and arm defects because of its size, versatility, ease of use, and reliability. The latissimus dorsi is a large, broad muscle that originates on the lower six thoracic and lumbar vertebrae, the lower four ribs, and the posterior ilium. It inserts on the intertubercular groove of the humerus and acts as an arm adductor. Its blood supply is from a single dominant pedicle in the axilla, the thoracodorsal artery. The muscle can be mobilized to include the entire muscle or

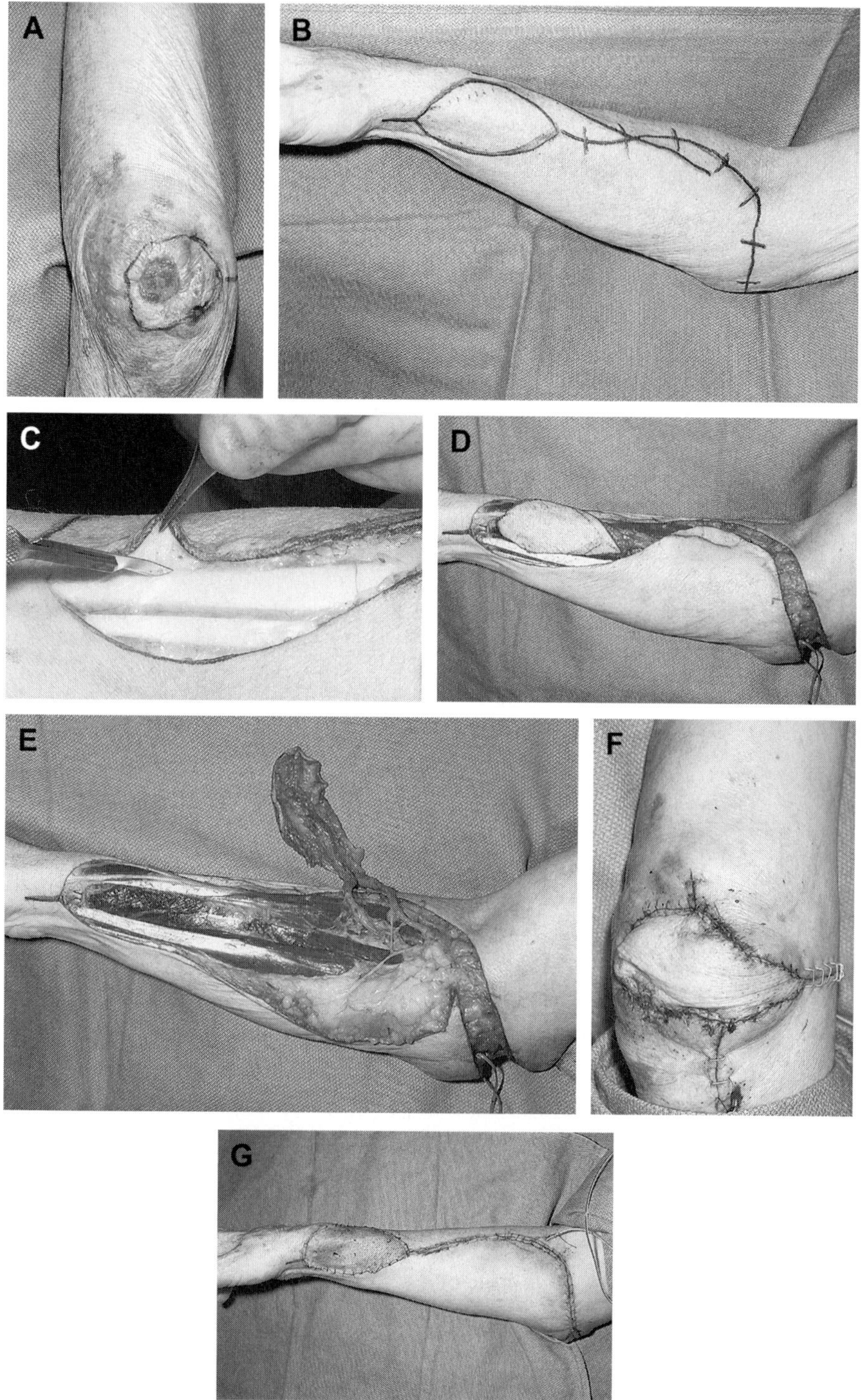

Fig. 2. The use of a radial forearm flight to cover a chronic posterior defect of the elbow. (*A*) An 84-year-old gentlemen with long-standing ulcer over the right elbow following trauma. (*B*) Flap is designed over the radial distal forearm and skin island is designed to include a branch of the cephalic vein. (*C*) Care is taken to preserve the paratenon during dissection over the FCR and brachioradialis to facilitate skin graft take over the donor site. (*D, E*) The cephalic vein and lateral antebrachial cutaneous nerve are included in flap dissection to improve venous outflow and provide sensation to the flap. (*F*) The flap is pedicled and inset into the donor site after subcutaneous transposition of the ulnar nerve. (*G*) The donor site is covered with an unmeshed split-thickness skin graft.

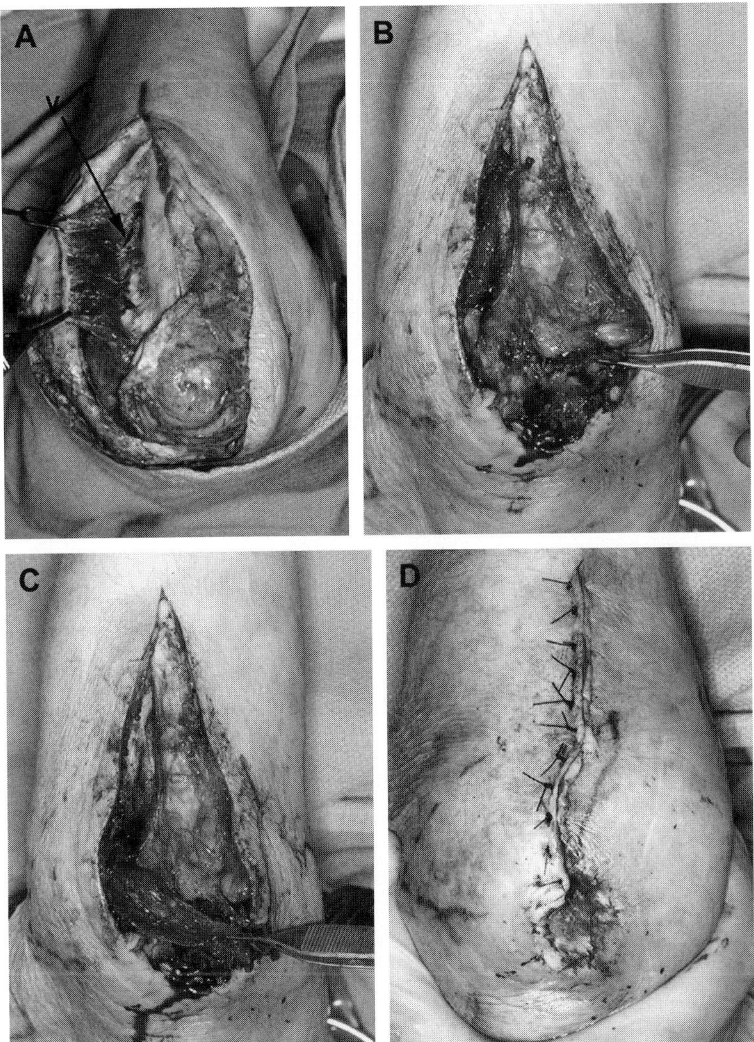

Fig. 3. The anconeus muscle flap may be used for the coverage of small traumatic defects around the elbow. (*A*) Flap elevation is performed most easily through separation of the muscle from its ulnar attachments and then identifying the vascular pedicle (v) running on the deep surface of the muscle. (*B*) Posterior traumatic elbow wound in a 26-year-old man with connection to joint. (*C, D*) Anconeus is mobilized to cover most proximal portion of wound and primary closure is performed over ulnar and distal aspect of wound.

just the anterior aspect of the muscle. A large skin paddle can be fashioned up to a size of 12 cm × 35 cm with primary closure of the donor site. When mobilized, the long, broad muscle rotates on its arc in the axilla and is tunneled into the arm. The flap can be used to cover large soft tissue defects in the arm or elbow and can reach as far as the midforearm. Additionally, the flap can be used as a functional muscle transfer in elbow flexorplasty or triceps plasty [46]. Its ease of use, large skin paddle size, minimal donor site morbidity

simplicity, large arc of rotation, versatility in functional muscle transfer, and reliability are the principal benefits of the latissimus dorsi flap [2,47–51].

Technique

The patient is placed in the lateral decubitus position, and the side and involved extremity are prepped from the neck to the iliac spine and from midline posteriorly to the nipple line anteriorly. A line is drawn for the incision several centimeters posterior to and parallel with the anterior border of the latissimus. If needed, the skin paddle is centered over the anterior muscle. The incision is carried down to the muscle fascia and dissection is made anteriorly to find the interval between the serratus anterior and the latissimus. The dissection is then carried distally and the distal origins are freed. The muscle is then mobilized proximally, bluntly freeing it from the teres major. The neurovascular pedicle is then identified and preserved. The thoracodorsal branch to the serratus anterior muscle is divided and the pedicle is dissected, dividing the circumflex scapular artery in the axilla if needed. The muscle is passed through a subcutaneous tunnel into the arm to the recipient site. The donor site is closed primarily over drains to reduce the development of a seroma, which can occur in as many as 30% of cases. Meticulous dissection and use of internal quilt suturing to coapt the deep dermis to the underlying muscle can also help prevent seroma formation [48,50,52].

Complications of the pedicled latissimus dorsi flap include significant distal flap loss, which occurs in as many as 38% of patients. Choudry and colleagues [43] found that distal flap loss was more common when extending the flap beyond the olecranon process, which may have been because of the more extensive distal dissection needed to harvest a long flap or from undue tension when securing the flap in place. Complete flap loss is less common. Minor complications include donor site seromas, skin graft loss, and hematomas. Using the latissimus flap as a free flap allows the bulk of the muscle to be centered over the defect and reduces distal flap loss (Fig. 4) [48,52].

Distant pedicled flaps

Historically, distant pedicled flaps raised from the chest or abdominal wall were commonly used for elbow coverage. They have now been nearly completely abandoned because of the multiple disadvantages with distant pedicled flaps, which include the need for a second operation to divide and inset the flap, prolonged hospital stay, and joint stiffness secondary to prolonged immobilization. The large array of local flaps, pedicled flaps, and free flaps has relegated the distant pedicled flap to use only in salvage situations when no better options for tissue coverage exist. Flaps that have been used for this purpose include the thoracoepigastric flap, based on the internal

mammary perforators; the lateral thoracic flap, based on the thoracodorsal or lateral thoracic artery; the external oblique fasciocutaneous flap, based on myocutaneous perforators; and the pectoralis major flap and the proximal-based rectus abdominis flap [53].

Free flaps

Microsurgical techniques have revolutionized the field of reconstructive surgery by allowing unlimited possibilities in soft tissue coverage. Free flaps can be made from any combination of muscle, bone, fascia, skin, viscera, or omentum as long as the flap is designed on a precise vascular pedicle and appropriate recipient vessels exist for anastomosis. Given a skilled microsurgical team, the flap failure rate should be less than 3% for blood vessels ranging from 0.5 to 2 mm. With this low failure rate and the ability to pick a donor site that matches the needs of the recipient tissues, free flap reconstruction is often a more attractive alternative than much simpler local flap coverage. Free flap reconstruction is also indicated in cases where local trauma excludes other possibilities, when external fixation precludes local flap use, or when single composite free-tissue transfer obviates the need for multistaged reconstruction. Donor site morbidity is also a factor that frequently favors distant tissue transfer because many donor sites can be closed primarily. Functional muscle transfers and neurotization of flaps increase the usefulness and versatility of free flap reconstruction. Given the numerous benefits to free flap reconstruction, many have called into question the traditional concept of the reconstructive ladder. Focus is placed on the individual surgeon's expertise, experience, and judgment in applying the correct reconstructive model to fit each patient. Form, function, and safety are emphasized, rather than simplicity of the initial procedure. Choice of flap is dictated by size of defect, donor site morbidity, and tissue defect [1,9,54–58].

Frequently used fasciocutaneous flaps include the anterolateral thigh, scapular, parascapular, and lateral arm flaps [59–61]. Some muscle flaps are preferred when infection is present or significant dead space needs to be filled. These may then be covered with a split-thickness skin graft or transferred with an overlying skin paddle. Potential donor sites for myocutaneous flaps include the latissimus dorsi, serratus anterior, rectus abdominis, or gracilis. Free neurotized muscle transfer is also possible to restore elbow flexion

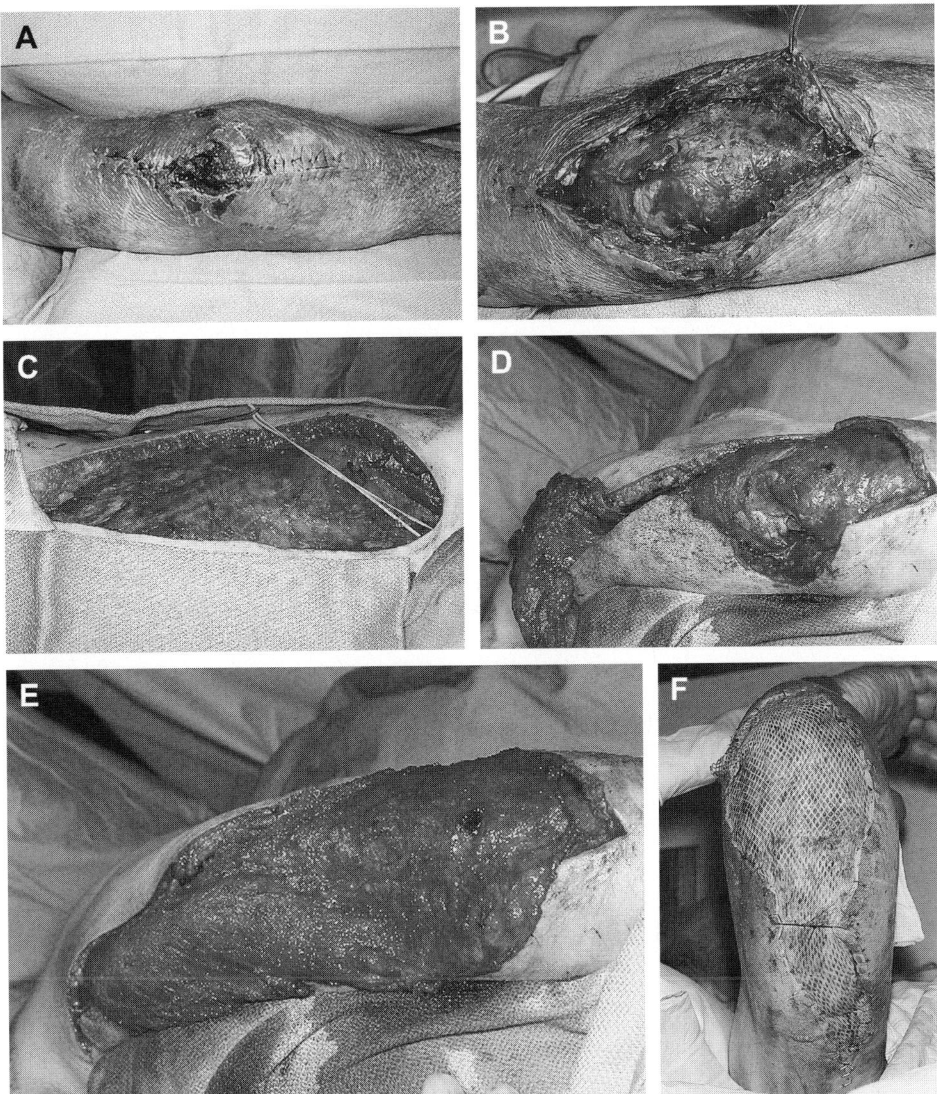

Fig. 4. (*A*) A 65-year-old renal transplant patient developed necrosis of posterior skin incision following placement of elbow prosthesis. (*B*) The elbow was debrided and then covered with the use of a pedicled latissimus dorsi flap. (*C*) Flap elevation was performed through a posterior lateral incision. (*D, E*) Division of the humeral insertion of the latissimus dorsi muscle allowed for transposition through an axillary skin tunnel and insetting over elbow. (*F*) Stable coverage was provided with the use of a split-thickness skin graft applied over the muscle; alternatively, a skin paddle may be taken with the latissimus dorsi muscle.

or finger flexion, as pioneered by Manktelow and McKee [62,63].

Composite flaps are used when tendon reconstruction or a vascularized bone graft is required. These can be useful for restoring function and allowing soft tissue and skin coverage simultaneously. Frequent sites for composite tissue harvest with bone include the fibula, based on the peroneal artery; the iliac crest, based on the deep circumflex iliac artery; the scapula, based on the circumflex scapular; or the radius, based on the radial artery [50,64–67].

The authors have found the anterior lateral thigh flap to provide great versatility for the coverage of elbow defects [59,68,69]. The anterior lateral thigh flap based on the lateral femoral circumflex artery may be harvested with a portion of the tensor fascia lata, vastus lateralis muscle, femoral cutaneous nerve, which allows the surgeon the potential to reconstruct skin deficits in addition to tendon deficits over the triceps insertion. The donor site may often be closed primarily (Fig. 5). Overall, free-tissue transfer to the elbow is facilitated by the large caliber of donor

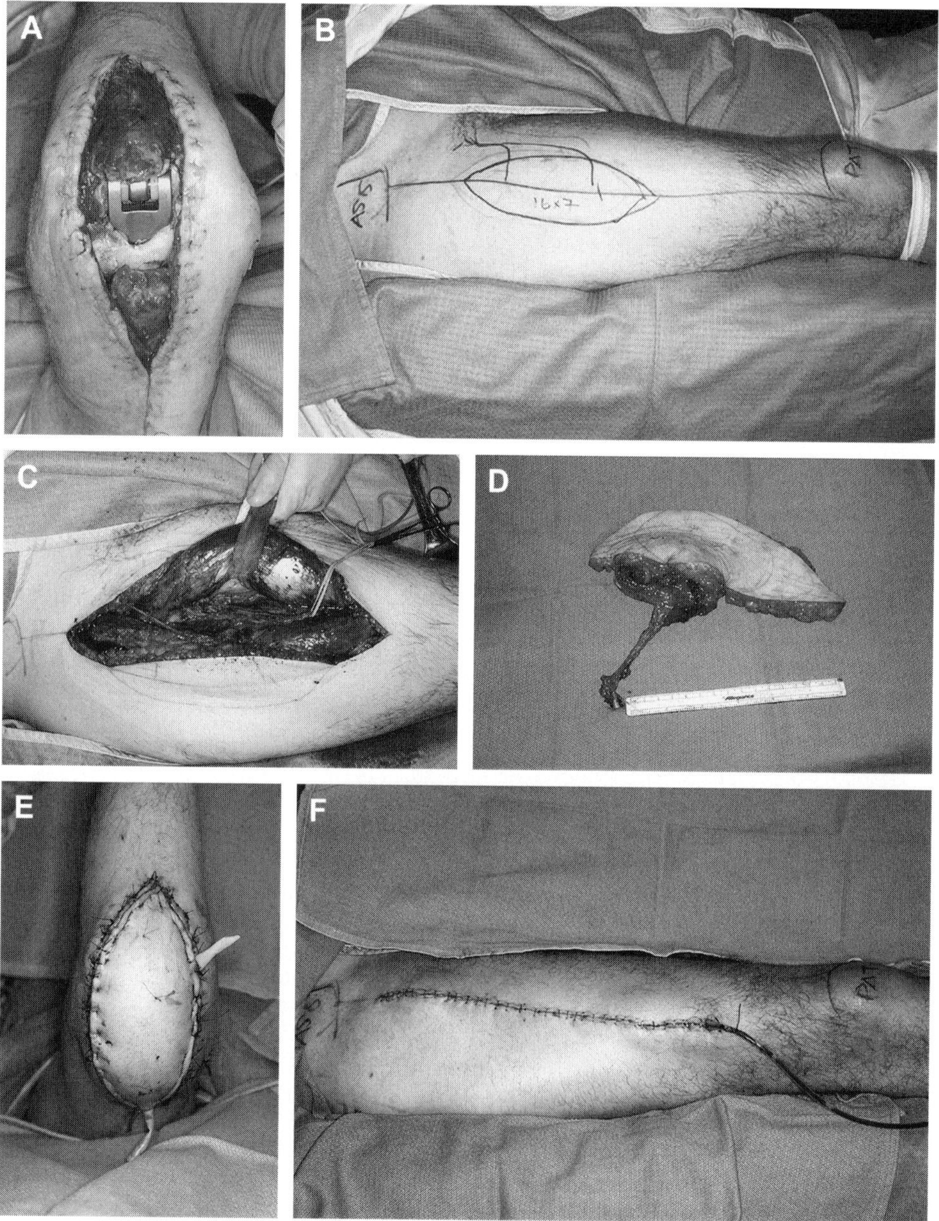

Fig. 5. (*A*) An exposed elbow prosthesis in a 66-year-old rheumatoid patient. (*B*) The patient was treated with a free anterior lateral thigh flap. The perforator for the flap can be found reliably at a point which lies halfway between the lateral margin of the patella and the superior iliac spine. (*C*) The lateral femoral circumflex artery is easily identified by retracting the rectus femoris muscle medially. (*D*) The flap is harvested with a cuff of vastus lateralis muscle to provide additional muscular tissue for dead space obliteration. (*E*) The donor site can be closed primarily. (*F*, *G*) The flap is then inset into the defect while the vessels are anastomosed end-to-side into the brachial system. (*H*, *I*) Final appearance of the flap.

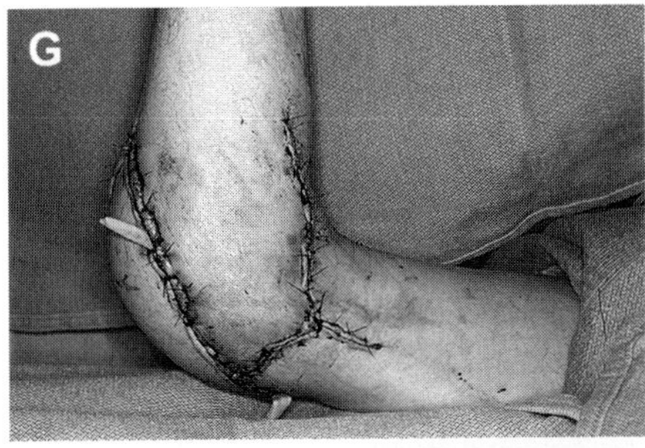
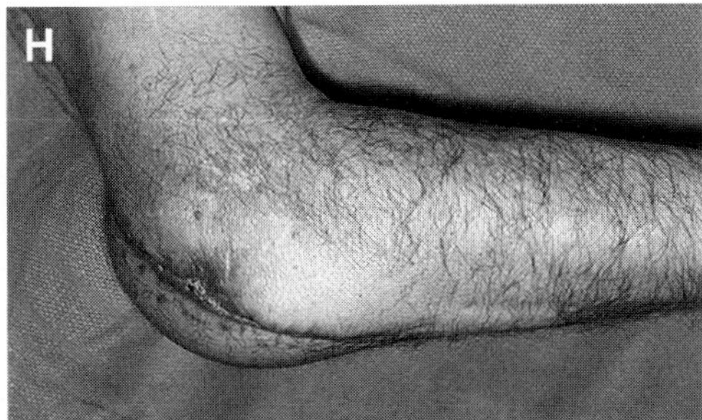
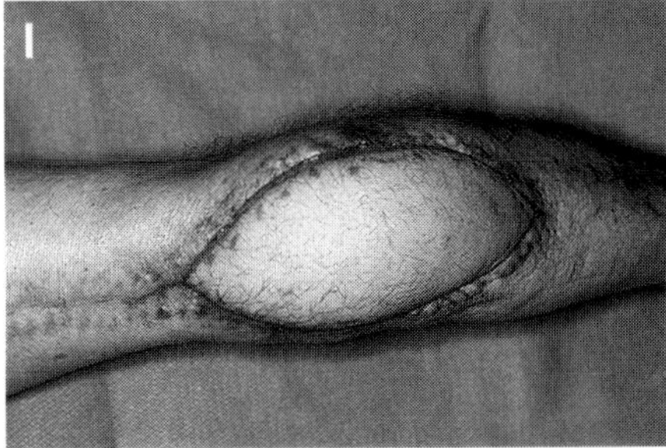

Fig. 5 (*continued*)

vessels within the antecubital fossa, with most flaps being placed end-to-side into the brachial artery and the recipient vein.

Outcomes studies

At present, no prospective outcome studies compare different flap types for elbow coverage; this deficiency is most likely due to the variability of wound size and concomitant injury. Hallock [70] described his experience with coverage options for traumatic wounds of the upper limb. He performed 16 local fascia flaps, 22 free flaps, 1 pedicled flap, and 1 local muscle flap. His preference for free flap coverage within this study is most likely attributable to the inclusion of hand injuries and only eight isolated elbow defects. Among the elbow injuries, he used five fascial flaps and three free flaps to obtain stable coverage [71]. Derderian and colleagues [71] similarly looked at their experience with exclusively free flaps to the entire upper extremity. Parascapular free flaps were the most prevalent flaps used (26%), with a flap failure rate of 9%.

Choudry and colleagues [43], in their retrospective comparative series of 99 flaps used specifically for the coverage of elbow defects, highlighted the usefulness of pedicled flaps (both muscular and fasciocutaneous) in the coverage of elbow defects. In this series, 66% of the flaps used for coverage were pedicled flaps, with the radial forearm flap being the most commonly used (37%). Sixteen percent of the wounds were initially covered with free-tissue transfers.

Within Choudry's series, only 10 cases required a second flap for elbow salvage. The pedicled latissimus flap was found to have the highest complication rate, with distal necrosis being the most frequent complication. Fourteen percent of the pedicled latissimus dorsi flaps were complicated by distal necrosis, wound breakdown, or failure at the reconstruction site, in comparison with the radial forearm and local fasciocutaneous flaps. In all cases of distal necrosis seen with the use of the pedicled latissimus dorsi muscle, the muscle was used to cover defects that had extended beyond the olecranon to the proximal ulna. The radial forearm flap had a significantly lower partial necrosis rate (4%) when compared with the pedicled latissimus flap for coverage of olecranon and proximal ulnar defects [43].

The pedicled latissimus dorsi flap has been a workhorse flap for coverage of the elbow, especially for large defects [52,72,73]. Its robust pedicle makes this flap reliable. However, the distal end of the flap can become tenuous if raised all the way to the origin of the muscle. This extended dissection becomes necessary if one

Table 1
Preferential treatment options for soft tissue coverage of the elbow

Defect size and location	Recommended coverage option
Small, proximal to olecranon	Local muscle flap or local fasciocutaneous flap
Large, proximal to olecranon	Pedicled LDF or free flap
Small, distal to olecranon	Local muscle flap or local fasciocutaneous flap
Large, distal to olecranon	Radial forearm flap or free flap

Abbreviation: LDF, Latissimus dorsi flap.

needs to cover defects that are distal to the olecranon process. Not only does one need to raise the entire muscle, but one may also need to put the flap on stretch to cover the entire defect. These conditions may contribute to the higher incidence of distal necrosis and wound breakdown.

The above findings have led the authors to rethink the use of pedicled latissimus dorsi flaps for defects extending over the proximal ulna. Stevanovic and colleagues [72] have recommended previously that the latissimus dorsi not be used routinely to cover defects more than 8 cm distal to the olecranon. For large defects, the authors now prefer free-tissue transfer, which allows easier positioning of the flap over the defect site. The radial forearm flap is also an excellent option for moderate-sized defects localized over the olecranon and proximal ulna. For smaller defects, the anconeus or radial forearm flap offers reliable soft tissue coverage. The authors' current treatment protocol is presented in Table 1.

References

[1] Geddes CR, Morris SF, Neligan PC. Perforator flaps: evolution, classification, and applications. Ann Plast Surg 2003;50:90–9.
[2] Sherman R. Soft-tissue coverage for the elbow. Hand Clin 1997;13:291–302.
[3] Ciresi KF, Mathes SJ. The classification of flaps. Orthop Clin North Am 1993;24:383–91.
[4] Breidenbach WC. Emergency free tissue transfer for reconstruction of acute upper extremity wounds. Clin Plast Surg 1989;16:505–14.
[5] Leininger BE, Rasmussen TE, Smith DL, et al. Experience with wound VAC and delayed primary closure of contaminated soft tissue injuries in Iraq. J Trauma 2006;61:1207–11.
[6] DeFranzo AJ, Argenta LC, Marks MW, et al. The use of vacuum-assisted closure therapy for the treatment of lower-extremity wounds with exposed bone. Plast Reconstr Surg 2001;108:1184–91.
[7] Arnold PG, Lovich SF, Pairolero PC. Muscle flaps in irradiated wounds: an account of 100 consecutive cases. Plast Reconstr Surg 1994;93:324–7.
[8] Moran SL, Illig KA, Green RM, et al. Free-tissue transfer in patients with peripheral vascular disease: a 10-year experience. Plast Reconstr Surg 2002;109: 999–1006.
[9] Kremer T, Bickert B, Germann G, et al. Outcome assessment after reconstruction of complex defects of the forearm and hand with osteocutaneous free flaps. Plast Reconstr Surg 2006;118(2):443–54.
[10] Germann G, Levin LS. Decision-making in reconstructive surgery (upper-extremity). Berlin: Springer; 2000 p. 181–221.
[11] Nahai F, Mathes SJ. Musculocutaneous flap or muscle flap and skin graft? Ann Plast Surg 1984; 12:199–203.
[12] DeLong WG Jr, Born CT, Wei SY, et al. Aggressive treatment of 119 open fracture wounds. J Trauma 1999;46:1049–54.
[13] Freshwater MF. Ten signs for successful skin grafting. Plast Reconstr Surg 1983;72:419–20.
[14] MacFarlane DF. Current techniques in skin grafting. Adv Dermatol 2006;22:125–38.
[15] Ratner D. Skin grafting. From here to there. Dermatol Clin 1998;16:75–90.
[16] Ablove RH, Howell RM. The physiology and technique of skin grafting. Hand Clin 1997;13:163–73.
[17] Rakel BA, Bermel MA, Abbott LI, et al. Split-thickness skin graft donor site care: a quantitative synthesis of the research. Appl Nurs Res 1998;11:174–82.
[18] Taylor GI, Caddy CM, Watterson PA, et al. The venous territories (venosomes) of the human body: experimental study and clinical implications. Plast Reconstr Surg 1990;86:185–213.
[19] Hudson DA. Some thoughts on choosing a Z-plasty: the Z made simple. Plast Reconstr Surg 2000;106: 665–71.
[20] Lister GD, Gibson T. Closure of rhomboid skin defects: the flaps of Limberg and Dufourmentel. Br J Plast Surg 1972;25:300–14.
[21] Lanzetta M, Bernier M, Chollet A, et al. The lateral forearm flap: an anatomic study. Plast Reconstr Surg 1997;99:460–4.
[22] Lamberty BG, Cormack GC. The forearm angiotomes. Br J Plast Surg 1982;35:420–9.
[23] Le Huec JC, Liquois F, Leger O, et al. A study of the fasciocutaneous vascularisation of the arm. Surgical applications. Surg Radiol Anat 1995;17:121–8.
[24] Orgill DP, Pribaz JJ, Morris DJ. Local fasciocutaneous flaps for olecranon coverage. Ann Plast Surg 1994;32:27–31.
[25] Parry SW, Ward JW, Mathes SJ. Vascular anatomy of the upper extremity muscles. Plast Reconstr Surg 1988;81:358–65.

[26] Heller F, Wei W, Wei FC. Chronic arterial insufficiency of the hand with fingertip necrosis 1 year after harvesting a radial forearm free flap. Plast Reconstr Surg 2004;114:728–31.

[27] Akpuaka FC. The radial recurrent fasciocutaneous flap for coverage of posterior elbow defects. Injury 1991;22:332–4.

[28] Culbertson JH, Mutimer K. The reverse lateral upper arm flap for elbow coverage. Ann Plast Surg 1987;18:62–8.

[29] Katsaros J, Schusterman M, Beppu M, et al. The lateral upper arm flap: anatomy and clinical applications. Ann Plast Surg 1984;12:489–500.

[30] Moffett TR, Madison SA, Derr JW Jr, et al. An extended approach for the vascular pedicle of the lateral arm free flap. Plast Reconstr Surg 1992;89:259–67.

[31] Lamberty BG, Cormack GC. The antecubital fascio-cutaneous flap. Br J Plast Surg 1983;36:428–33.

[32] Ohtsuka H, Imagawa S. Reconstruction of a posterior defect of the elbow joint using an extensor carpi radialis longus myocutaneous flap: case report. Br J Plast Surg 1985;38:238–40.

[33] Jones BM, O'Brien CJ. Acute ischaemia of the hand resulting from elevation of a radial forearm flap. Br J Plast Surg 1985;38:396–7.

[34] Bardsley AF, Soutar DS, Elliot D, et al. Reducing morbidity in the radial forearm flap donor site. Plast Reconstr Surg 1990;86:287–92.

[35] Hulsbergen-Kruger S, Muller K, Partecke BD. [Donor site defect after removal of free and pedicled forearm flaps: functional and cosmetic results]. Handchir Mikrochir Plast Chir 1996;28:70–5 [in German].

[36] Suominen S, Ahovuo J, Asko-Seljavaara S. Donor site morbidity of radial forearm flaps. A clinical and ultrasonographic evaluation. Scand J Plast Reconstr Surg Hand Surg 1996;30:57–61.

[37] Timmons MJ, Missotten FE, Poole MD, et al. Complications of radial forearm flap donor sites. Br J Plast Surg 1986;39:176–8.

[38] Richardson D, Fisher SE, Vaughan ED, et al. Radial forearm flap donor-site complications and morbidity: a prospective study [see comment]. Plast Reconstr Surg 1997;99:109–15.

[39] Calderon W, Chang N, Mathes SJ. Comparison of the effect of bacterial inoculation in musculocutaneous and fasciocutaneous flaps. Plast Reconstr Surg 1986;77:785–94.

[40] Chang N, Mathes SJ. Comparison of the effect of bacterial inoculation in musculocutaneous and random-pattern flaps. Plast Reconstr Surg 1982;70:1–10.

[41] Rohrich RJ, Ingram AE Jr. Brachioradialis muscle flap: clinical anatomy and use in soft-tissue reconstruction of the elbow. Ann Plast Surg 1995;35:70–6.

[42] Eshima I, Mathes SJ, Paty P. Comparison of the intracellular bacterial killing activity of leukocytes in musculocutaneous and random-pattern flaps. Plast Reconstr Surg 1990;86:541–7.

[43] Choudry UH, Moran SL, Li S, et al. Soft-tissue coverage of the elbow: an outcome analysis and reconstructive algorithm. Plast Reconstr Surg 2007;119.

[44] Mathes SJ, Nahia F. Classification of the vascular anatomy of muscles: experimental and clinical correlation. Plast Reconstr Surg 1981;67:177.

[45] Schmidt CC, Kohut GN, Greenberg JA, et al. The anconeus muscle flap: its anatomy and clinical application. J Hand Surg [Am] 1999;24:359–69.

[46] Stern PJ, Neale HW, Gregory RO, et al. Latissimus dorsi myocutaneous flap for elbow flexion. J Hand Surg [Am] 1982;7:25–30.

[47] Axer A, Segal D, Elkon A. Partial transposition of the latissimus dorsi. A new operative technique to restore elbow and finger flexion. J Bone Joint Surg Am 1973;55:1259–64.

[48] Bostwick J 3rd, Nahai F, Wallace JG, et al. Sixty latissimus dorsi flaps. Plast Reconstr Surg 1979;63:31–41.

[49] Pruzansky M, Kelly M, Weinberg H. Latissimus dorsi musculocutaneous flap for elbow extension. J Surg Oncol 1991;47:62–6.

[50] Angrigiani C, Grilli D, Siebert J. Latissimus dorsi musculocutaneous flap without muscle. Plast Reconstr Surg 1995;96:1608–14.

[51] Brones MF, Wheeler ES, Lesavoy MA. Restoration of elbow flexion and arm contour with the latissimus dorsi myocutaneous flap. Plast Reconstr Surg 1982;69:329–32.

[52] Chang LD, Goldberg NH, Chang B, et al. Elbow defect coverage with a one-staged, tunneled latissimus dorsi transposition flap. Ann Plast Surg 1994;32:496–502.

[53] Winspur I. Distant flaps. Hand Clin 1985;1:729–39.

[54] Daniel RK, Weiland AJ. Free tissue transfers for upper extremity reconstruction. J Hand Surg [Am] 1982;7:66–76.

[55] Godina M. Early microsurgical reconstruction of complex trauma of the extremities. Plast Reconstr Surg 1986;78:285–92.

[56] Liebermann-Meffert D. The greater omentum. Anatomy, embryology, and surgical applications. Surg Clin North Am 2000;80:275–93.

[57] Hultman CS, Carlson GW, Losken A, et al. Utility of the omentum in the reconstruction of complex extraperitoneal wounds and defects: donor-site complications in 135 patients from 1975 to 2000. Ann Surg 2002;235:782–95.

[58] Ullmann Y, Fodor L, Ramon Y, et al. The revised "reconstructive ladder" and its applications for high-energy injuries to the extremities. Ann Plast Surg 2006;56:401–5.

[59] Chen HC, Tang YB, Mardini S, et al. Reconstruction of the hand and upper limb with free flaps based on musculocutaneous perforators. Microsurgery 2004;24:270–80.

[60] Kremer T, Bickert B, Germann G, et al. Outcome assessment after reconstruction of complex defects of

the forearm and hand with osteocutaneous free flaps. Plast Reconstr Surg 2006;118:443–54.

[61] Yildirim S, Taylan G, Eker G, et al. Free flap choice for soft tissue reconstruction of the severely damaged upper extremity. J Reconstr Microsurg 2006;22:599–609.

[62] Manktelow RT, Zuker RM, McKee NH. Functioning free muscle transplantation. J Hand Surg [Am] 1984;9:32–9.

[63] Manktelow RT, McKee NH. Free muscle transplantation to provide active finger flexion. J Hand Surg [Am] 1978;3:416–26.

[64] Hamilton SG, Morrison WA. The scapular free flap. Br J Plast Surg 1982;35:2–7.

[65] Urbaniak JR, Koman LA, Goldner RD, et al. The vascularized cutaneous scapular flap. Plast Reconstr Surg 1982;69:772–8.

[66] Zhou G, Qiao Q, Chen GY, et al. Clinical experience and surgical anatomy of 32 free anterolateral thigh flap transplantations [comment]. Br J Plast Surg 1991;44:91–6.

[67] Rose PS, Shin AY, Bishop AT, et al. Vascularized free fibula transfer for oncologic reconstruction of the humerus. Clin Orthop Relat Res 2005;438:80–4.

[68] Muneuchi G, Suzuki S, Ito O, et al. Free anterolateral thigh fasciocutaneous flap with a fat/fascia extension for reconstruction of tendon gliding surface in severe bursitis of the dorsal hand [report]. Ann Plast Surg 2002;49(3):312–6.

[69] Wei FC, Jain VM, Celik N, et al. Have we found an ideal soft-tissue flap? An experience with 672 anterolateral thigh flaps. Plast Reconstr Surg 2002;109:2219–26.

[70] Hallock GG. The utility of both muscle and fascia flaps in severe upper extremity trauma. J Trauma 2002;53:61–5.

[71] Derderian CA, Olivier WAM, Baux G, et al. Microvascular free-tissue transfer for traumatic defects of the upper extremity: a 25-year experience. J Reconstr Microsurg 2003;19:455–61.

[72] Stevanovic M, Sharpe F, Itamura JM. Treatment of soft tissue problems about the elbow. Clin Orthop Relat Res 2000;370:127–37.

[73] Pierce TD, Tomaino MM. Use of the pedicled latissimus muscle flap for upper-extremity reconstruction. J Am Acad Orthop Surg 2000;8:324–31.

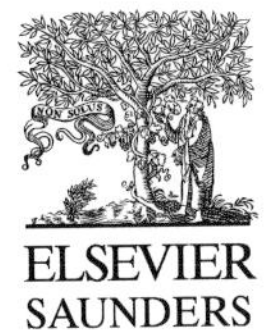

ORTHOPEDIC
CLINICS
OF NORTH AMERICA

Orthop Clin N Am 39 (2008) 265–268

Index

Note: Page numbers of article titles are in **boldface** type.

A

Anconeus flap, in soft tissue coverage of elbow, 255

Arthroplasty
    radial head, for radial head fractures, 179–181
    total elbow
        in distal humerus fracture management, 194–197
        in prosthetic replacement for distal humerus fractures, 205–207

Arthroscopy, in chronic lateral elbow instability management, 227

Axial fasciocutaneous flaps, in soft tissue coverage of elbow, 254

B

Biceps, rupture of, distal, **237–249.** See also *Distal biceps rupture.*

Bryan-Morrey approach, to prosthetic replacement for distal humerus fractures, 205

C

Children
    fractures in
        lateral condyle, 167–169
        medial epicondyle, 169–170
        transphyseal elbow, 170
    lateral condyle fractures in, 167–169
    medial epicondyle fractures in, 169–170
    physeal elbow fractures in, **163–171**
    supracondylar fractures in, **163–171**
    transphyseal elbow fractures in, 170

Chronic lateral elbow instability, **221–228**
    clinical presentation of, 223
    fractures associated with, 222–223
    imaging studies of, 224
    mechanism of, 221
    pathoanatomy of, 221–222
    physical examination of, 223–224
    treatment of, 224–227

arthroscopy in, 227
    results of, 227
    surgical, 224–227

Chronic medial elbow instability, **213–219**
    anatomy relevant to, 213
    biomechanics of, 213–214
    clinical examination of, 214
    mechanism of injury, 214
    radiography of, 215
    sequelae of, 217–218
    treatment of
        nonoperative, 215
        operative, 215–217
        rehabilitation in, 217

Coronoid, stabilization of, 146–147

D

Dislocation(s), elbow, acute, **155–161.** See also *Elbow, dislocations of, acute.*

Distal biceps rupture, **237–249**
    biomechanical studies of, 245–247
    causes of, 237–238
    classification of, 239
    clinical evaluation of, 238
    complete, treatment of, 239
    demographics of, 237
    partial, treatment of, 239
    treatment of, 239–244
        complications of, 244–245
        Endobutton in, 243
        interference screw in, 243–244
        single anterior incision in, 242
        suture anchor in, 242–243
        two-incision technique in, 239–242

Distal humerus fractures, **187–200**
    classification of, 187–188
    clinical evaluation of, 188
    epidemiology of, 187
    management of
        complications of, 197–198

Distal (*continued*)
    definitive stabilization of distal segment and
        articular surface in, 193–194
    heterotropic ossification after, 198
    implant biomechanics in, 192
    metaphyseal compression and definitive
        proximal fixation in, 194
    nonoperative, 188
    nonunion after, 198
    operative, 188–194
    outcomes of, 197–198
    postoperative, 194
    prosthetic replacement in, **201–212**
        Bryan-Morrey approach to, 205
        classification of, 202
        clinical evaluation in, 202
        complications of, 209–210
        epidemiology of, 201–202
        hemiarthroplasty in, 207–208
        olecranon osteotomy in, 205
        outcomes of, 208–209
        paratricipital approach to, 203
        postoperative management in, 207
        surgical approach to, 202–203
        total elbow arthroplasty in, 205–207
        triceps splitting approach to, 203–205
    provisional plate application in, 193
    reduction and provisional fixation of
        articular surface in, 192–193
    surgical, 188–192
    total elbow arthroplasty in, 194–197
    transolecranon osteotomy in, 188–190
    TRAP approach in, 191–192
    triceps sparing in, 190
    triceps splitting in, 190–191

Distal pedicled flaps, in soft tissue coverage of
    elbow, 258

E

Elbow, **141–154**
    anatomy of, 141–144, 229–230
        capsuloligamentous, 142–144
        muscles, 142
        osteoarticular, 141–142
    arthroplasty of, total, in distal humerus
        fracture management, 194–197
    biomechanics of, 144–152
    dislocations of, acute, **155–161**
        causes of, 155
        classification of, 156
        diagnosis of, 156
        injuries associated with, 156–157
        pathophysiology of, 155–156
        treatment of, 157–159
            authors' preferred, 160–161
            complications of, 159–160
            rehabilitation in, 159
            results of, 159
            surgical, 157–159
    flexion-extension of, 144–145
    fractures of
        in children, **163–171**
            evaluation of, 163
                radiography in, 163–164
        ossification of, 163–164
    instability of
        chronic lateral, **221–228.** See also *Chronic
            lateral elbow instability.*
        chronic medial, **213–219.** See also *Chronic
            medial elbow instability.*
    joint forces of, 152
    kinematics of, 144–146
    osseous stabilization of, 146–148
        coronoid, 146–147
        olecranon, 147–148
        proximal radius, 148
    pronation-supination of, 145–146
    soft tissue coverage of, **251–264**
        flaps in, 253–261. See also *Flap(s), in soft
            tissue coverage of elbow.*
        general principles of, 251
        patient assessment for, 251–252
        primary closure in, 252
        skin grafting for, 252–253
        surgical planning for, 252
        timing of, 251–252
    soft tissue stabilization of, 148–151
        lateral collateral ligament complex in,
            149–150
        medial collateral ligament complex in,
            148–149
        muscles in, 150–151

Endobutton, in distal biceps rupture management,
    243

F

Flap(s). See also specific types, e.g., *Local random
    flaps.*
    in soft tissue coverage of elbow,
        253–261
        axial fasciocutaneous flaps, 254
        local random flaps, 253–254
        outcomes of, 261–262
        pedicle muscle flaps, 255–261
        radial forearm island flap, 254–255
    terminology related to, 253

Fracture(s)
    chronic lateral elbow instability–related,
      222–223
    distal humerus, **187–200.** See also *Distal*
      humerus fractures.
        prosthetic replacement in, **201–212.** See also
          Distal humerus fractures, management of,
          prosthetic replacement in.
    in children
      lateral condyle, 167–169
      medial epicondyle, 169–170
      transphyseal elbow, 170
    lateral condyle, in children, 167–169
    olecranon, **229–236.** See also *Olecranon*
      fractures.
    physeal elbow, in children, **163–171**
    radial head, treatment of, **173–185.** See also
      Radial head fractures, treatment of.
    supracondylar, in children, **164–167**

Free flaps, in soft tissue coverage of elbow,
    258–261

H

Hemiarthroplasty, in prosthetic replacement for
    distal humerus fractures, 207–208

Heterotropic ossification, distal humerus fracture
    management and, 198

I

Instability, elbow
    chronic lateral, **221–228.** See also *Chronic*
      lateral elbow instability.
    chronic medial, **213–219.** See also *Chronic*
      medial elbow instability.

Interference screw, in distal biceps rupture
    management, 243–244

K

Kinematic(s), of elbow, 144–146

L

Lateral collateral ligament complex, stabilization
    of, 149–150

Lateral condyle fractures, in children, 167–169

Lateral ligament complex repair, for radial head
    fractures, 181

Latissimus dorsi myocutaneous pedicle flap, in
    soft tissue coverage of elbow, 255–258

LCDC plate fixation. See *Limited-contract dynamic*
    compression (LCDC) plate fixation.

Limited-contract dynamic compression (LCDC)
    plate fixation, in olecranon fracture
    management, 233–234

Local random flaps, in soft tissue coverage of
    elbow, 253–254

M

Medial collateral ligament complex, stabilization
    of, 148–149

Medial epicondyle fractures, in children, 169–170

Muscle(s), of elbow
    anatomy of, 142
    stabilization of, 150–151

N

Nonunion, distal humerus fracture management
    and, 198

O

Olecranon, stabilization of, 147–148

Olecranon fractures, **229–236**
    classification of, 230
    diagnosis of, 230–231
      clinical examination in, 231
      imaging in, 231
      patient history in, 230–231
      radiography in, 231
    mechanism of injury, 230
    treatment of, 231–234
      complications of, 234–235
      LCDC plate fixation in, 233–234
      outcomes of, 235–236
      rehabilitation in, 235
      results of, 235–236
      tension band wire in, 231–233

Olecranon osteotomy, in prosthetic replacement
    for distal humerus fractures, 205

Olecranon process, anatomy of, 229–230

Open reduction and internal fixation (ORIF)
    for distal humerus fractures, 192–193
    for radial head fractures, 176–177

ORIF. See *Open reduction and internal fixation*
    (ORIF).

Osteotomy, transolecranon, in distal humerus
    fracture management, 188–190

P

Pedicle muscle flaps, in soft tissue coverage
of elbow, 255–261
anconeus flap, 255
distal pedicled flaps, 258
free flaps, 258–261
latissimus dorsi myocutaneous pedicle flap,
255–258

Physeal elbow fractures, in children,
163–171

Prosthesis(es), in distal humerus fractures
management, **201–212.** See also *Distal humerus
fractures, management of, prosthetic replacement
in.*

Proximal radius, stabilization of, 148

R

Radial forearm island flap, in soft tissue coverage
of elbow, 254–255

Radial head arthroplasty, for radial head
fractures, 179–181

Radial head excision, for radial head fractures,
177–179

Radial head fractures
classification of, 175
imaging of, 174–175
mechanism of injury, 173–174
signs and symptoms of, 173–174
treatment of, **173–185**
complications of, 182
lateral ligament complex repair in, 181
nonoperative, 175
open reduction and internal fixation in,
176–177
operative, 175–181
radial head arthroplasty in, 179–181
radial head excision in, 177–179
rehabilitation in, 181–182
surgical, 175–176

Radiography
in elbow fracture evaluation, 163–164
in olecranon fractures evaluation, 231
of chronic medial elbow instability, 215

Radius, proximal, stabilization of, 148

Rehabilitation
for acute elbow dislocations, 159
for chronic medial elbow instability, 217
in olecranon fracture management, 235
in radial head fracture management, 181–182

Rupture, distal biceps, **237–249.** See also *Distal
biceps rupture.*

S

Soft tissue, elbow coverage with, **251–264.** See also
Elbow, soft tissue coverage of.

Soft tissue stabilization, of elbow, 148–151

Supracondylar fractures, in children, **164–167**

T

Tension band wire, in olecranon fracture
management, 231–233

Total elbow arthroplasty
in distal humerus fracture management,
194–197
in prosthetic replacement for distal humerus
fractures, 205–207

Transolecranon osteotomy, in distal humerus
fractures management, 188–190

Transphyseal elbow fractures, in children, 170

Triceps reflecting anconeus pedicle (TRAP)
approach, in distal humerus fracture
management, 191–192

Triceps sparing, in distal humerus fracture
management, 190

Triceps splitting, in distal humerus fracture
management, 190–191